Free Radial Artery Forearm Flap for Head and Neck Reconstruction
A Color Atlas

Free Radial Artery Forearm Flap for Head and Neck Reconstruction
A Color Atlas

Editors

Girish N Amlani
MS(General Surgery) MCh(Plastic Surgery)
Honorary Head and Neck Reconstructive Surgeon
Shri NM Virani Wockhardt Hospital
Rajkot, Gujarat, India

Dipen D Patel
MS(General Surgery) MCh(Surgical Oncology)
Consultant Surgical Oncologist and Head
Department of Surgical Oncology
Shri NM Virani Wockhardt Hospital
Rajkot, Gujarat, India

Foreword
Santosh Raibagkar

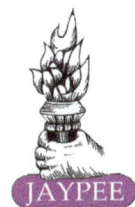

JAYPEE BROTHERS MEDICAL PUBLISHERS
The Health Sciences Publisher
New Delhi | London

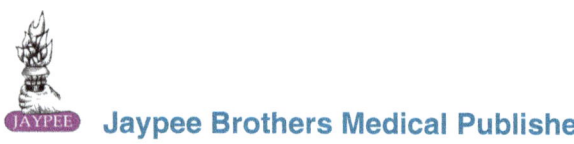
Jaypee Brothers Medical Publishers (P) Ltd

Headquarters
Jaypee Brothers Medical Publishers (P) Ltd
4838/24, Ansari Road, Daryaganj
New Delhi 110 002, India
Phone: +91-11-43574357
Fax: +91-11-43574314
E-mail: jaypee@jaypeebrothers.com

Overseas Office
JP Medical Ltd
83 Victoria Street, London
SW1H 0HW (UK)
Phone: +44 20 3170 8910
Fax: +44 (0)20 3008 6180
E-mail: info@jpmedpub.com

Website: www.jaypeebrothers.com
Website: www.jaypeedigital.com

© 2020, Jaypee Brothers Medical Publishers

The views and opinions expressed in this book are solely those of the original contributor(s)/author(s) and do not necessarily represent those of editor(s) of the book.

All rights reserved. No part of this publication may be reproduced, stored or transmitted in any form or by any means, electronic, mechanical, photocopying, recording or otherwise, without the prior permission in writing of the publishers.

All brand names and product names used in this book are trade names, service marks, trademarks or registered trademarks of their respective owners. The publisher is not associated with any product or vendor mentioned in this book.

Medical knowledge and practice change constantly. This book is designed to provide accurate, authoritative information about the subject matter in question. However, readers are advised to check the most current information available on procedures included and check information from the manufacturer of each product to be administered, to verify the recommended dose, formula, method and duration of administration, adverse effects and contraindications. It is the responsibility of the practitioner to take all appropriate safety precautions. Neither the publisher nor the author(s)/editor(s) assume any liability for any injury and/or damage to persons or property arising from or related to use of material in this book.

This book is sold on the understanding that the publisher is not engaged in providing professional medical services. If such advice or services are required, the services of a competent medical professional should be sought.

Every effort has been made where necessary to contact holders of copyright to obtain permission to reproduce copyright material. If any have been inadvertently overlooked, the publisher will be pleased to make the necessary arrangements at the first opportunity. The **CD/DVD-ROM** (if any) provided in the sealed envelope with this book is complimentary and free of cost. **Not meant for sale.**

Inquiries for bulk sales may be solicited at: jaypee@jaypeebrothers.com

Free Radial Artery Forearm Flap for Head and Neck Reconstruction: A Color Atlas

First Edition: **2020**

ISBN: 978-93-89776-77-5

Dedicated to
Our parents, teachers and family

Foreword

I was overjoyed, when I was asked to write a brief foreword from Dr Girish N Amlani and Dr Dipen D Patel for this book titled *Free Radial Artery Forearm Flap for Head and Neck Reconstruction: A Color Atlas*. Dr Girish is a dedicated surgeon and I appreciate the amount of hard work he puts in, anything he works on especially microsurgery. His team has done a very good job. I am happy to go through the Color Atlas of Free Radial Artery Forearm Flap for Head and Neck Reconstruction with complete description and depiction of variety of cases.

I think this is the only color atlas having excellent illustrations demonstrating technique in detail. It will be very useful for those interested in head and neck reconstruction.

To summarize, a Color Atlas of Free Radial Artery Forearm Flap is surely a book to treasure for every one who is interested in reconstructive surgery. I wish them a very bright future.

Santosh Raibagkar
MS MCh(Plastic Surgery)
Consultant Plastic Surgeon and
Ex-Professor of Plastic Surgery
AMC MET Medical College
LG General Hospital
Ahmedabad, Gujarat, India

Preface

After completing MCh (Plastic Surgery) in 1995, I Dr Girish N Amlani joined Shri Nathalal Parekh Cancer Hospital and Research Center, Rajkot, Gujarat as honorary plastic surgeon and did more than 3000 head and neck reconstructions till 2014. I have done more than 1000 head and neck reconstructions working with other oncosurgeons of Rajkot, Gujarat. I underwent training in microsurgery under the renowned, Dr S Rajasabapathy at Ganga Hospital, Coimbatore, Tamil Nadu. He taught me finer aspects of microsurgery. Dr Dipen D Patel did MCh (Surgical Oncology) in June 2016 and joined Shri NM Virani Wockhardt Hospital, Rajkot, Gujarat, India. We are sharing our experience of free radial artery forearm flap, a recent workforce of head and neck reconstruction, as a color atlas.

Girish N Amlani
Dipen D Patel

Acknowledgments

We express our indebtedness to Dr Udyan Vyas, Dr Santosh Raibagkar, Dr Jayvirsinh Jhala, Dr Nitin Tolia, Dr Ramkrishna N, anesthetist team, Dr Rajesh Radadia, Dr Dhaval Karoriya, Dr Tejas Chauhan, Dr Rajesh Sakaria, Dr Bhavik Bhuva, and other staff members of Shri NM Virani Wockhardt Hospital, Rajkot, Gujarat, India.

We thank Khorakiwala family for running MA Yojna program for cancer patients. This has proved as boon to them.

We offer our profound gratitude to Shri Jitendar P Vij (Group Chairman), Mr Ankit Vij (Managing Director), Mr MS Mani (Group President), Ms Chetna Malhotra Vohra (Associate Director—Content Strategy), Ms Pooja Bhandari (Production Head), Ms Savleen Kaur (Development Editor) and Mr Sharad Patel (Commissioning Editor, Ahmedabad Branch) of M/s Jaypee Brothers Medical Publishers (P) Ltd, New Delhi, India for their constant support in publishing this color atlas.

Contents

1. Introduction 1
2. Historical Perspective 2
3. Advantages and Disadvantages..3
4. Anatomy..4
5. Preoperative Preparation 6
6. Operative Steps of Free Radial Artery Forearm Flap 7
7. Postoperative Care 38
8. Case Studies 39
9. Complications 85

Suggested Reading 86

Index 87

CHAPTER 1

Introduction

The radial artery forearm flap was one of the first free flaps to be described. Free radial artery forearm flap is used to replace external skin and internal mucosal lining and has become workhorse for head and neck cancer reconstruction.

Free radial artery forearm flap has very thin and pliable skin. Large flap of 30 × 15 cm size can be harvested. Multiple skin islands[1] can be planned. We can harvest flap with lateral antebrachial nerve for sensate flap particularly for tongue reconstruction.[2]

Radius bone can be incorporated in flap for osteocutaneous[3,4] reconstruction, but free fibula is preferred. Palmaris longus[5-8] tendon can be incorporated in flap for sling for lower lip reconstruction. Free radial artery forearm flap can be easily tubed for pharyngeal reconstruction.

It has got large, long, reliable and constant vascular pedicle. Head and neck resection and harvesting of free radial artery forearm flap can be done simultaneously. It has got large distal end of vessel to be used as a flow—through flap for and additional flap to be attached distally.

REFERENCES

1. Sakai S, Soeda S, Endo T, Ishii M, Uchiumi E. A compound radial artery forearm flap for the reconstruction of lip and chin defect. Br J Plast Surg. 1989;42(3):337-8.
2. Stock W, Muhlhauer W, Biemer E. The neurovascular forearm island flap. Z Plast Chir. 1981;5:158-65.
3. Sautar DS, Widdowson WP. Immediate reconstruction of mandible using a vascularized segment of radius. Head Neck Surg. 1986;8:232-46.
4. Villaret DB, Futran NA. The indications and outcomes in the use of osteocutaneous radial forearm free flap. Head Neck. 2003;25:475-81.
5. Ndou R, Gangata H, Mitchell B, Ngcongo T, Louw G. The frequency of absence of palmaris longus in a South African population of mixed race. Clin Anat. 2010;23(4):437-42.
6. Sadove RC, Luce EA, McGrath PC. Reconstruction of the lower lip and chin with the composite radial forearm palmaris longus free flap. Plast Reconstr Surg. 1991;88(2):209-14.
7. Jeng SF, Kuo YR, Wei FC, Su CY, Chien CY. Total lower lip reconstruction with a composite radial forearm palmaris longus tendon flap: a clinical series. Plast Reconstr Surg. 2004;113(1):19-23.
8. Agarwal P. Absence of the palmaris longus tendon in Indian population. Indian J Orthop. 2010;44(2):212-5.

CHAPTER 2

Historical Perspective

The radial artery forearm flap was developed in China. Dr Yang Guofan[1] and Dr Gao Yuzhi described anatomical studies in 1978. First free radial artery forearm flap was performed in Shenyang Military Hospital and afterwards they published clinical study of 60 cases in 1981. The radial artery forearm flap is type C fasciocutaneous flap, nicknamed as Chinese flap.

The pedicle flap based on the retrograde flow from the palmar arch was described by Biemer and Lu in 1981. Muhlbauer[2] and Soutar advocated restricting flap harvesting on the palmar forearm for improving cosmetic outcome in 1982 and 1986. Fenton[3] covered flexor carpi radialis tendon with its muscle for better graft take up in 1985. Hallock[4] converted donor site into a linear scar by using tissue expansion in 1998.

REFERENCES

1. Yang GF, Chen B, Gao Y. Forearm free skin flap transplantation. Natl Med J China. 1981;61:139-42.
2. Muhlbauer W, Herndl E, Stock W. The forearm flap. Plast Reconstr Surg. 1982;70:336-44.
3. Fenton OM, Roberts JO. Improving the donor site of the radial forearm flap. Br J Plast Surg. 1985;38:504-5.
4. Hallock GG. Refinement of the radial forearm flap donor site using skin expansion. Plast Reconstr Surg. 1988;81:21-5.

CHAPTER 3

Advantages and Disadvantages

■ ADVANTAGES

The radial artery forearm flap can be harvested with large skin paddle.[1] The flap can be taken with forearm skin leaving behind 3 cm of strip on ulnar border of forearm. It is very reliable flap with success rate of 98% to 100% as it has numerous perforator and constant anatomy.[2] It has get long and sizeable pedicle and can reach to opposite neck for anastomosis. The radial artery forearm flap is very thin and pliable,[1] so it is very useful for defects of buccal mucosa and tongue reconstruction.

■ DISADVANTAGES

The donor site morbidities such as exposure of flexor tendons and poor donor site cosmesis are major drawbacks of the radial artery forearm flap.[3,4] Suprafascial dissection reduces morbidity of flap dramatically and grafted donor site remains unsightly on long run.

■ REFERENCES

1. Jeremić JV, Nikolić ŽS. Versatility of radial forearm free flap for intraoral reconstruction. Srp Arh Celok Lek. 2015;143(5-6):256-60.
2. Soutar DS, McGregor IA. The radial forearm flap in intraoral reconstruction: the experience of 60 consecutive cases. Plast Reconstr Surg. 1986;78:1-8.
3. Bardsley AF, Soutar DS, Elliot D, Batchelor AG. Reducing morbidity in the radial forearm flap donor site. Plast Reconstr Surg. 1990;86:287-92.
4. Gaukroger MC, Langdon JD, Whear NM, Zaki GA. Repair of the radial forearm flap donor site with a full-thickness graft. Int J Oral Maxillofac Surg. 1994;23:205-8.

CHAPTER

4

Anatomy

SURGICAL ANATOMY

Anatomy of Radial Artery in Forearm[1] (Fig. 1)

The radial artery is smaller than the ulnar artery and appears a more direct continuation of the brachial artery. Radial artery[2] starts 1 cm distal to the flexion crease of the elbow. Radial artery descends along the lateral side of the forearm from the medial side of the neck of the radius to the wrist. Radial artery is accompanied by paired venae comitantes. The radial artery lies on tendon of biceps, supinator, the distal attachment of pronator teres, the radial head of flexor digitorum superficialis, flexor pollicis longus, pronator quadratus and the lower end of the radius. Brachioradialis is lateral to the radial artery throughout its length. Pronator teres is medial to the radial artery proximally and flexor carpi radialis lies medially in distal portion.

The radial artery[3] has septocutaneous perforators in lateral intermuscular septum to overlying forearm skin. The perforators form arcade of vessels superficial to the deep fascia. The radial artery is accompanied by two venae comitantes draining into the medial cubital vein. The cephalic vein drains the flap through superficial subcutaneous veins. Either or both systems can be used for venous drainage of the radial artery forearm flap.

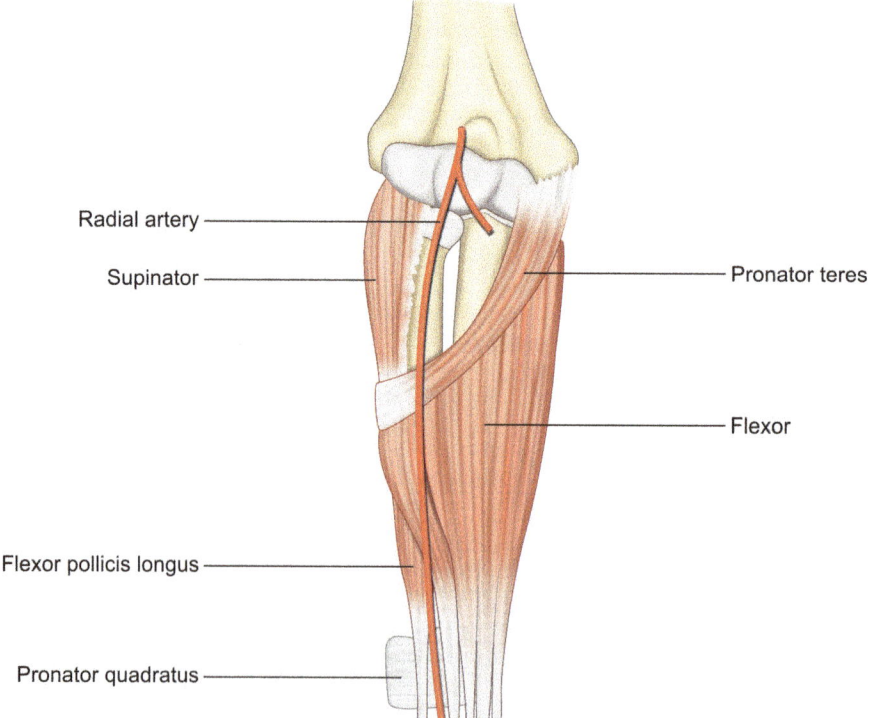

Fig. 1: Anatomy of radial artery in forearm.

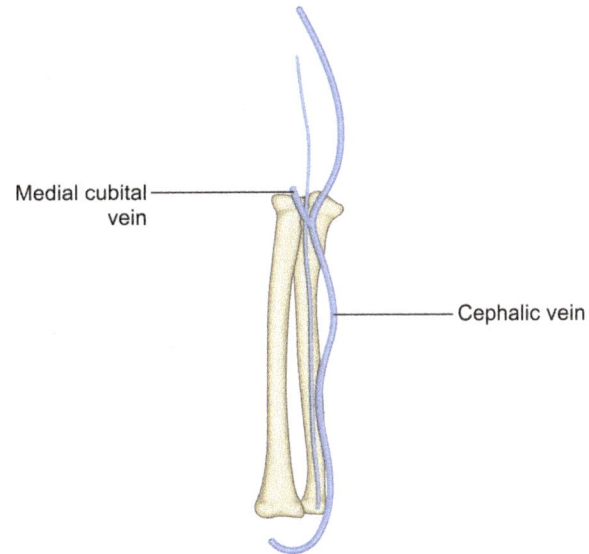

Fig. 2: Anatomy of cephalic vein.

Anatomy of Cephalic Vein[1] (Fig. 2)

The cephalic vein forms over the anatomical snuff box from the radial end of the dorsal venous plexus. Cephalic vein curves proximally around the radial side of the forearm to gain its ventral aspect. It receives veins from the both aspects of the forearm. The medial cubital vein, a branch distal to the elbow diverges proximomedially to reach the basilic vein. The medial cubital vein is joined by a branch from deep veins.

REFERENCES

1. Gray's Anatomy: Fortieth Edition. pp. 852-3.
2. Cormack GC, Lamberty BGH 1994. The Arterial Anatomy of Skin Flap Edinburgh: Churchill Livingstone.
3. Salmon M 1994 Anatomic Studies. In: Taylor GI, Razaboni RM (Eds), Book 1: Arteries of the Muscles of the Extremities and the Trunk. Book 2: Arterial Anastomotic Pathways of the Extremities. St Louis MO: Quality Medical Publishing.

CHAPTER 5

Preoperative Preparation

We prefer nondominant limb for the harvest of radial artery forearm flap. Upper limb having better cephalic vein should be preferred. Chemotherapeutic injection causes vasculitis and thrombosis of cephalic vein.

Allen's test should be done and intravenous cannulation should be avoided in operative limb.

MODIFIED ALLEN'S TEST[1,2]

The patients should clench their fist for 30 seconds first than the radial artery and ulnar artery are occluded at the wrist level. The patient should open fist and the pallor is observed over the thenar eminence. The pressure our ulnar artery is released and return of rubor is noted. Allen's test is negative, if rubor returns in less than 6 seconds, the test is equivocal in 7–11 seconds and test is positive if rubor does not return in 12 seconds.

Color Doppler and CT angiography show path of radial artery and intactness of palmar arch. If palmar arch is not patent, we go for radial artery forearm flap in opposite limb or other flap. In our series, radial artery has diameter of 1.9 mm to 3.5 mm.

REFERENCES

1. Allen EV. Thromboangiitis obliterans: methods of diagnosis of chronic arterial lesions distal to the wrist with illustrative cases. Am J Med Sci. 1929;178(3):165-89.
2. Jarvis MA, Jarvis CL, Jones PR, Spyt TJ. Reliability of Allen's test in selection of patient for radial artery harvest. Ann Thorac Surg. 2000;70(4):1362-5.

CHAPTER 6

Operative Steps of Free Radial Artery Forearm Flap

■ OPERATIVE STEPS[1-3]

Tourniquet is applied. 250 mm Hg pressure is preferred. Defect is measured. Flap is marked of same size and shape of the defect. We try to keep our distal margin of flap 2 cm proximal to wrist line, but if necessary, we can extend up to wrist line. Flap is usually extended radial to cephalic vein. Proximal incision from flap is kept up to elbow line in lazy S manner. Flap is dissected from radial side up to ulnar border of brachioradialis in suprafascial plane.[4] We preserve one of the three branches of sensory radial nerve. Flap is dissected from ulnar side up to radial border of flexor carpi radialis tendon in suprafascial plane. Cephalic vein is ligated with ligaclips. Radial artery and two venae comitantes are ligated with ligaclips. Flap is raised from distal to proximal in subfascial plane between flexor carpi radialis and brachioradialis tendons. All branches of radial artery and venae comitantes are ligated with ligaclips. We should avoid injury to paratenon of tendons of forearm. Cephalic vein is dissected up to elbow. Radial artery is dissected up to its origin from brachial artery, usually 1.5 cm distal to elbow line. Venae comitantes are dissected. One of the venae comitantes is larger. The large venae comitant is preferred for anastomosis. The smaller venae comitant is ligated with ligaclips. Antebrachial nerve is dissected whenever we are planning sensate flap. Tourniquet is released and hemostasis is completed. Now neck vessels are prepared for anastomosis under loupe magnification or under microscope. facial artery and superior thyroid artery are preferred. We can use transverse cervical artery, external carotid artery and opposite facial artery for anastomosis. For dissecting radial artery, we cut digastric muscle and tendon as blood flow is better in proximal part of facial artery. Facial vein, common facial vein, superior thyroid vein, lingual vein, external jugular vein and internal jugular vein can be used for venous anastomosis. We prefer use of small veins for end-to-end anastomosis rather than end-to-side anastomosis in internal jugular vein. We prefer two venous anastomosis. Now cephalic vein is ligated proximally with ligaclips and divided with micro scissors. Radial artery is clipped with ligaclips distal to origin from brachial artery and divided.[5-7] Larger venae comitant is clipped and divided. Flap is brought in the neck. Complete inset is given. Now facial artery or any donor artery is sutured to radial artery with 8-0 prolene or 9-0 ethilon. Venae comitant is sutured to common facial or superior thyroid vein with 10-0 ethilon. Cephalic vein is anastomosed to external jugular vein with 8-0 prolene or 9-0 ethilon. We give 4000 units heparin intravenously after arterial anastomosis. A solution of 100 mL normal saline with 30 plain lignocaine and one ampoule of papaverine is used as a spray during anastomosis. Hemostasis is done. Drain is kept in neck away from sites of anastomosis. Neck is closed layerwise. Wound is closed in forearm with 3-0 ethilon. Split thickness skin graft is taken from thigh and placed over donor site of flap.

INSTRUMENTS FOR MICROSURGICAL RECONSTRUCTION

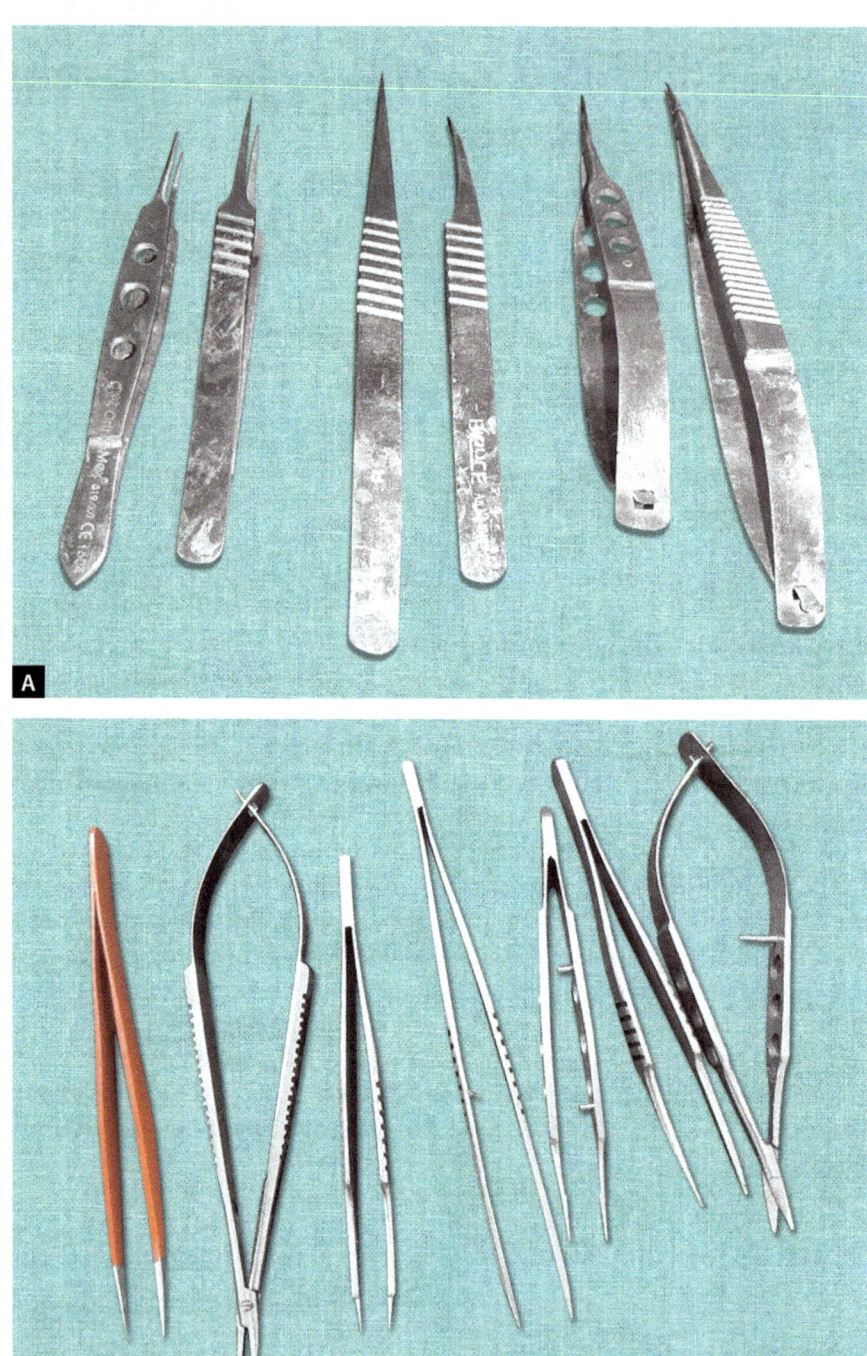

Figs. 1A and B: Instruments for microsurgery.

Operative Steps of Free Radial Artery Forearm Flap

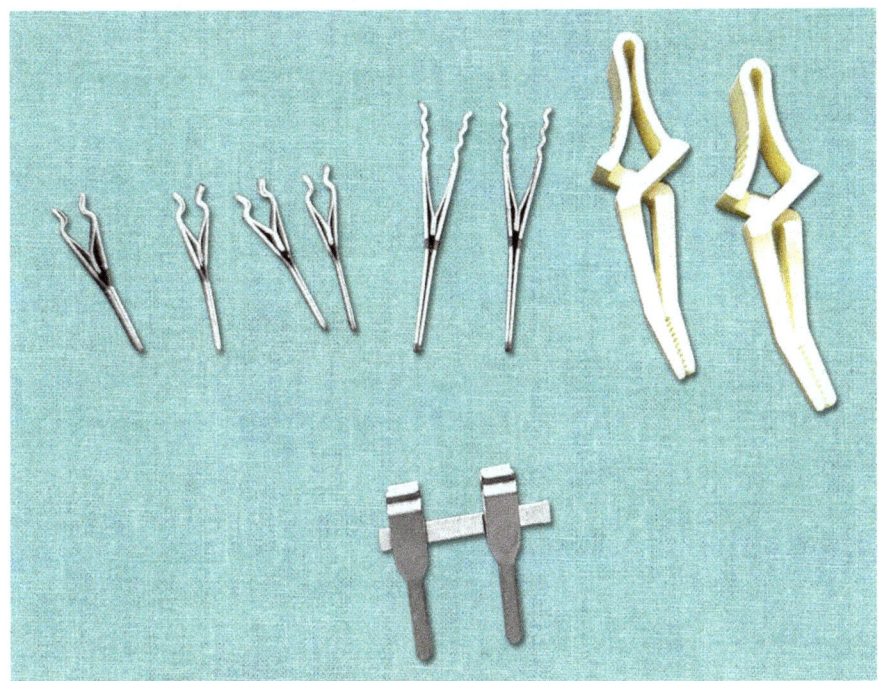

Fig. 2: Clamps for microsurgery.

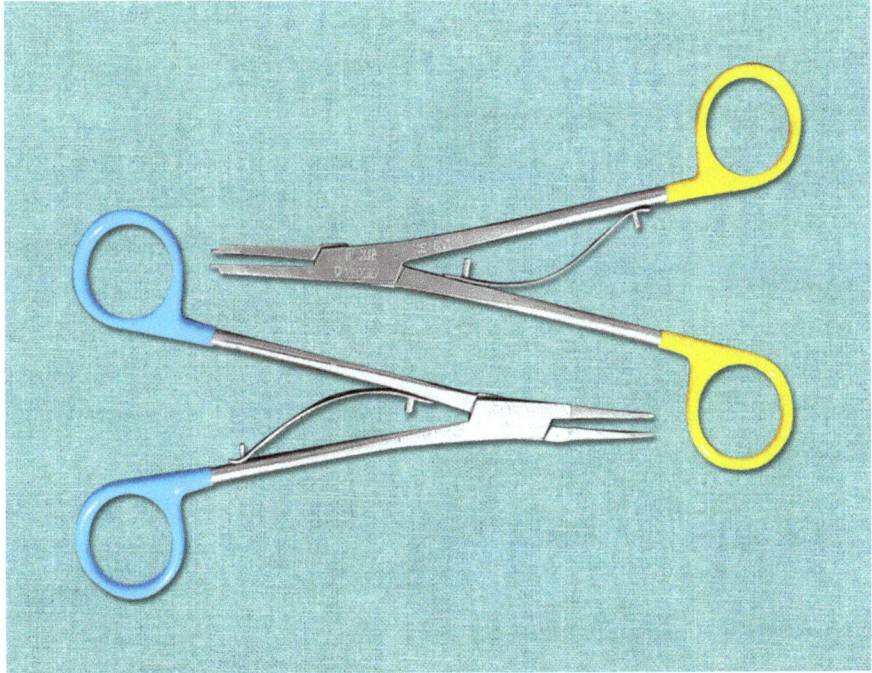

Fig. 3: Ligaclip applicators.

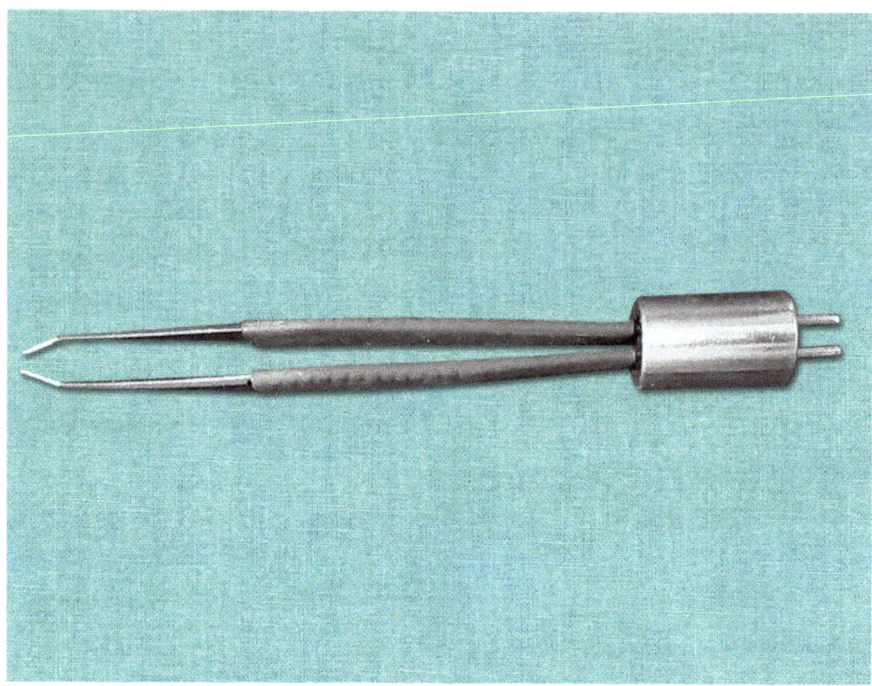

Fig. 4: Fine bipolar cautery forceps.

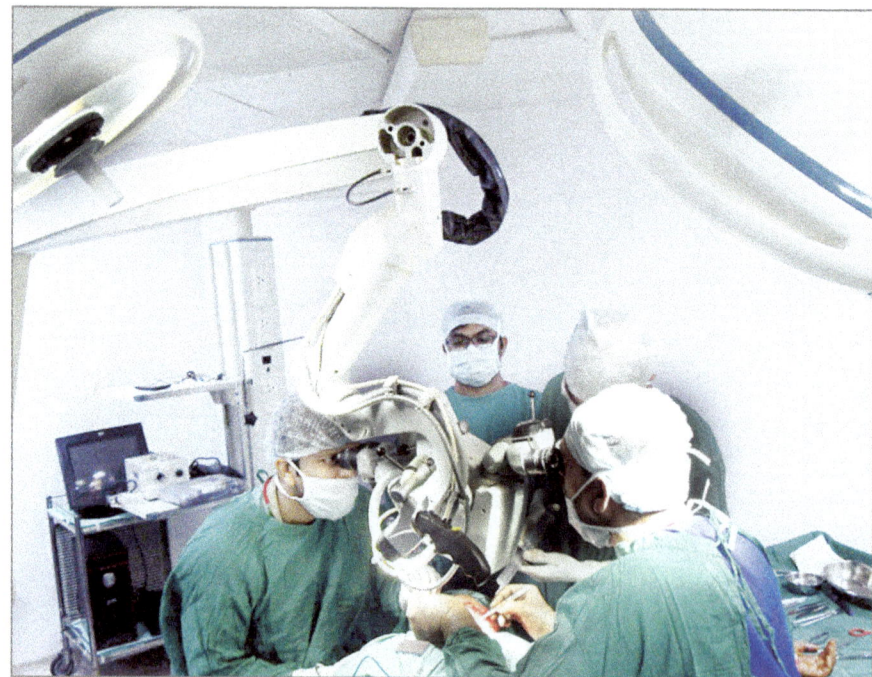

Fig. 5: Operative microscope: diploscope.

Operative Steps of Free Radial Artery Forearm Flap

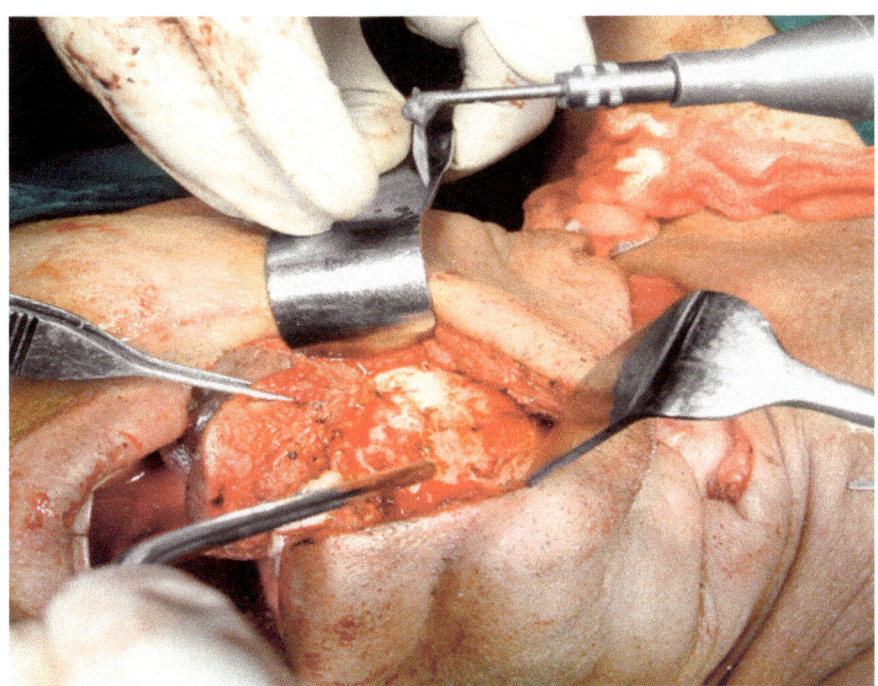

Fig. 6: Use of oscillating saw for marginal mandibulectomy.

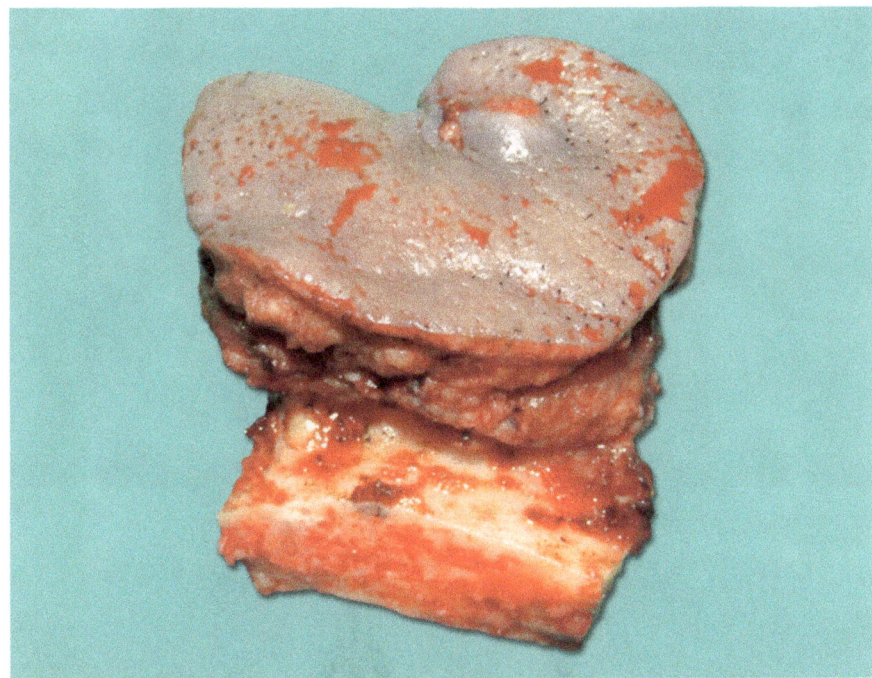

Fig. 7: Specimen.

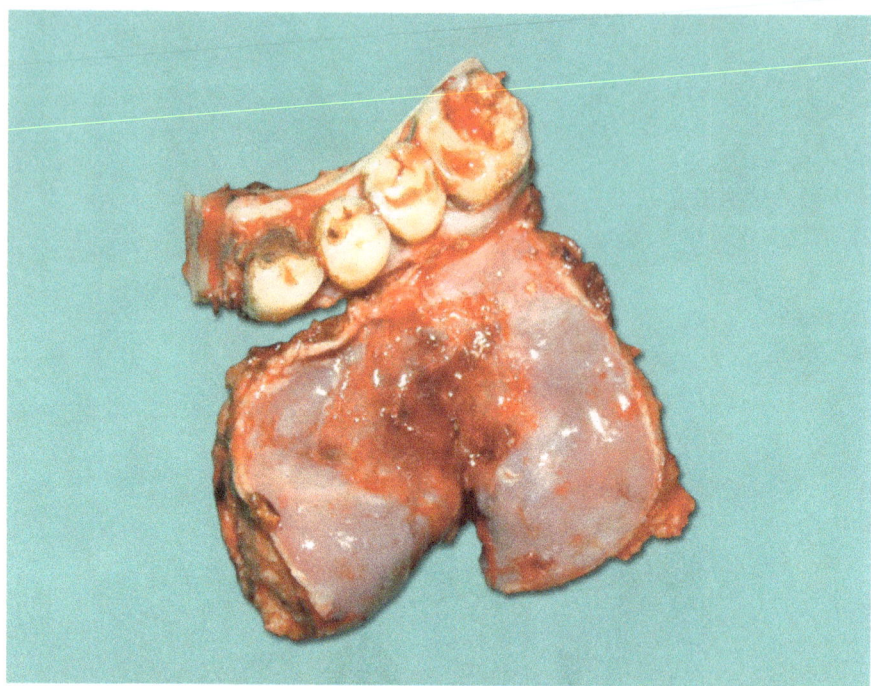

Fig. 8: Excised lesion with marginal mandibulectomy.

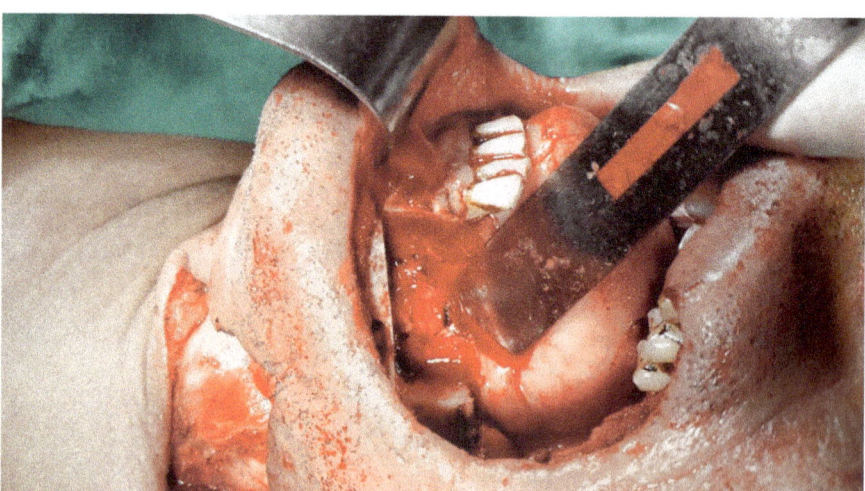

Fig. 9: Defect after marginal mandibulectomy.

Operative Steps of Free Radial Artery Forearm Flap

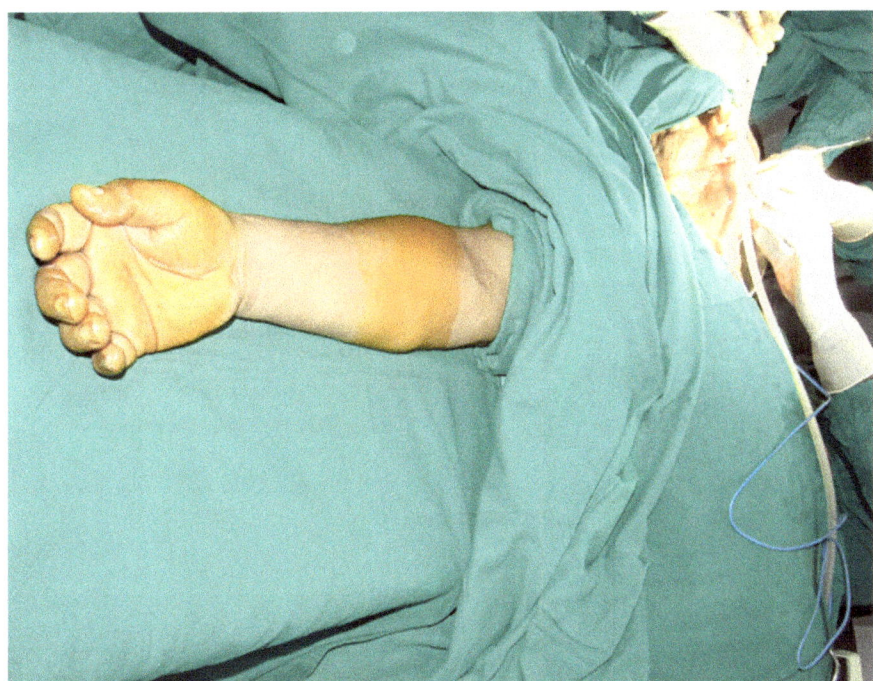

Fig. 10: Arm is extended and tourniquet is raised.

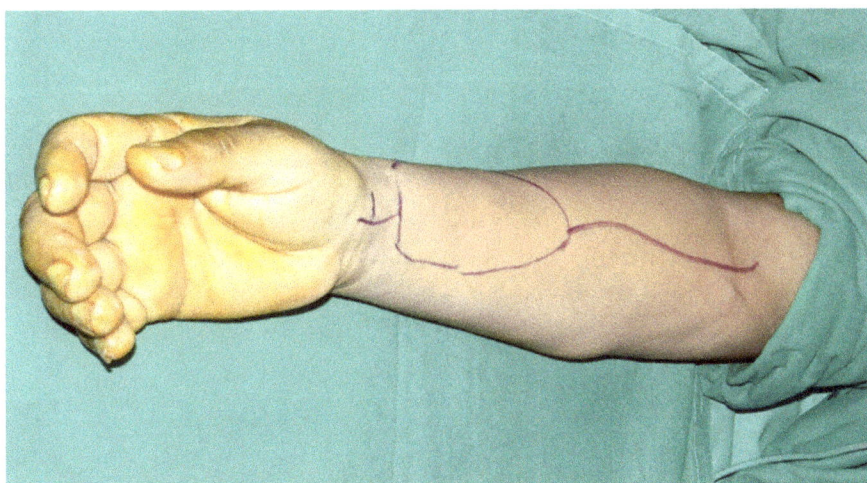

Fig. 11: Flap is marked.

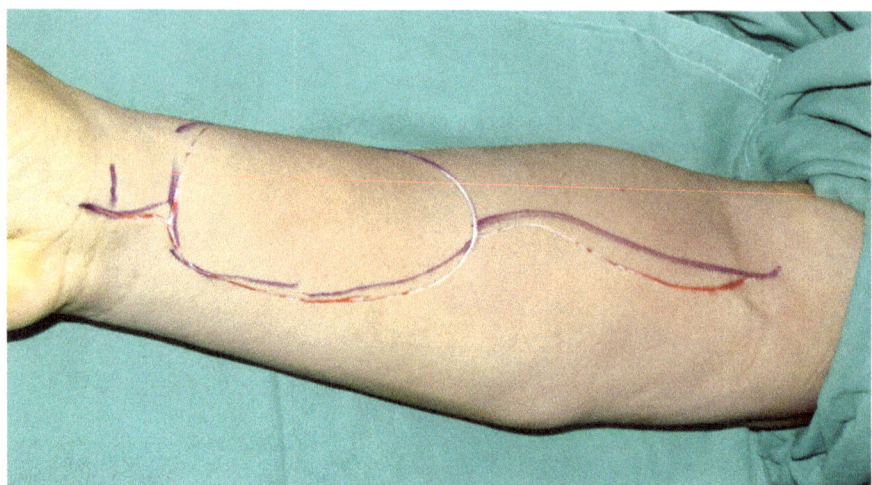

Fig. 12: Incision is kept.

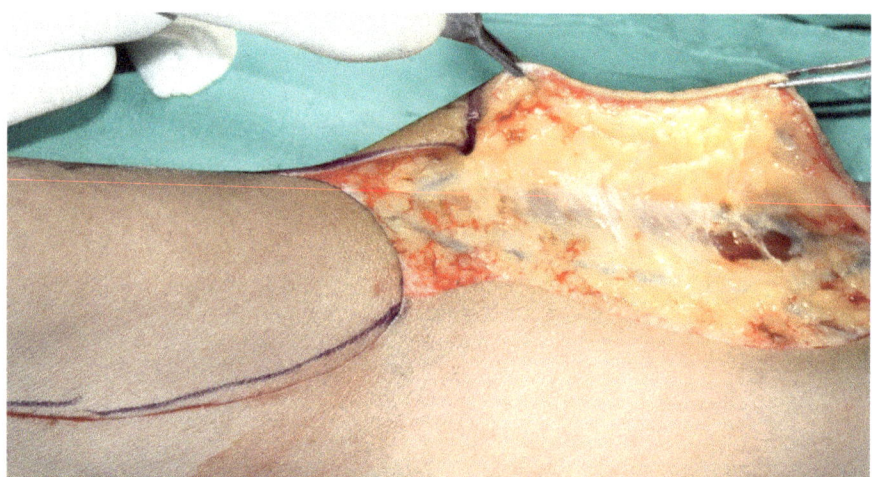

Fig. 13: Flaps are raised.

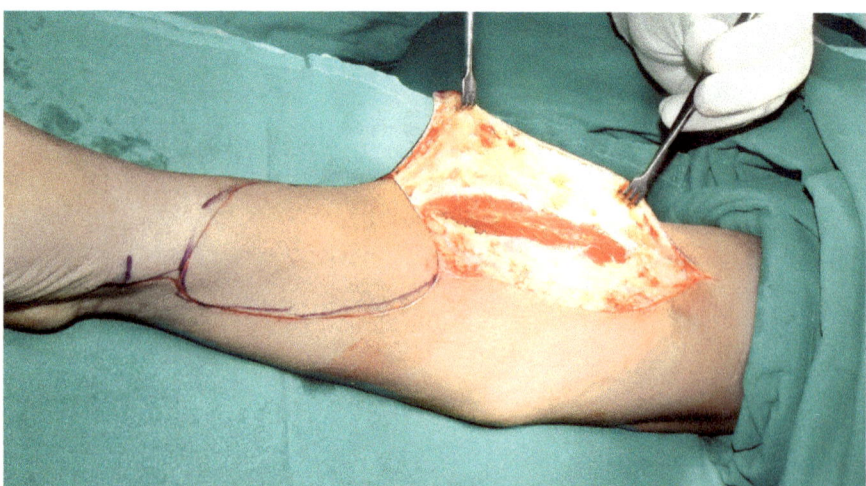

Fig. 14: Proximally cephalic vein and radial artery with venae comitantes are dissected up to elbow.

Operative Steps of Free Radial Artery Forearm Flap

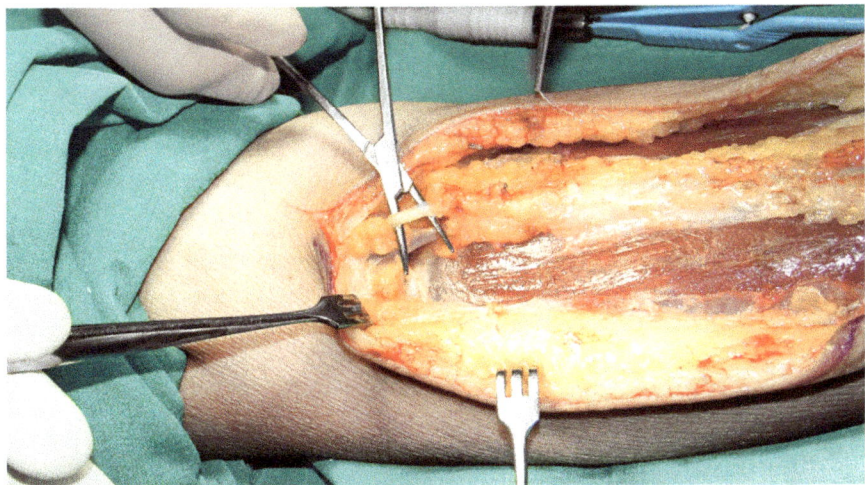

Fig. 15: Lateral antebrachial nerve and cephalic vein are seen.

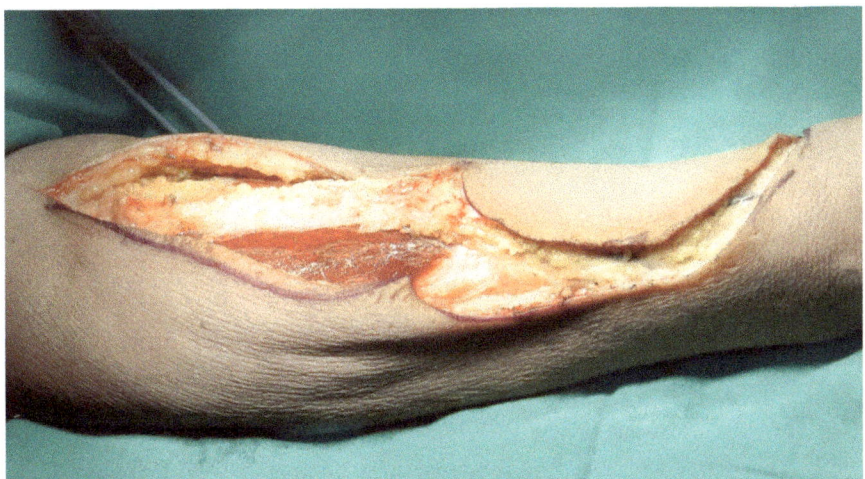

Fig. 16: Flap is dissected from radial side in suprafascial plane up to ulnar border of brachioradialis.

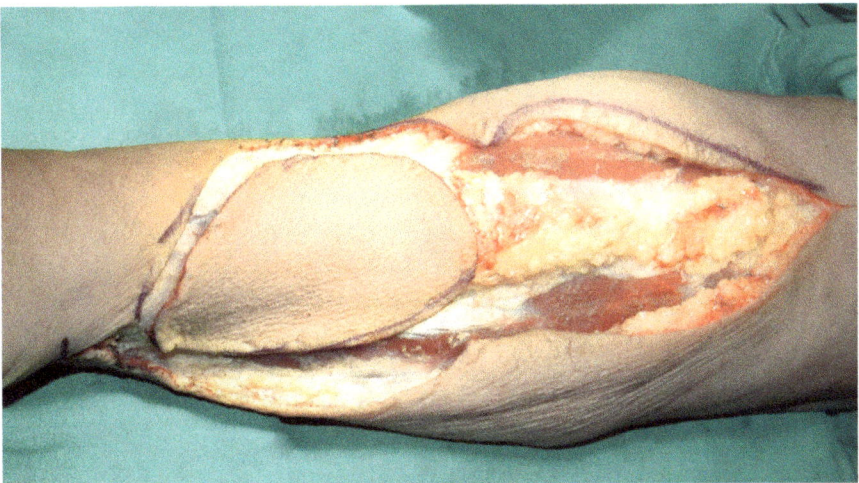

Fig. 17: Flap is dissected from ulnar side in suprafascial plane up to radial border of flexor carpi radialis.

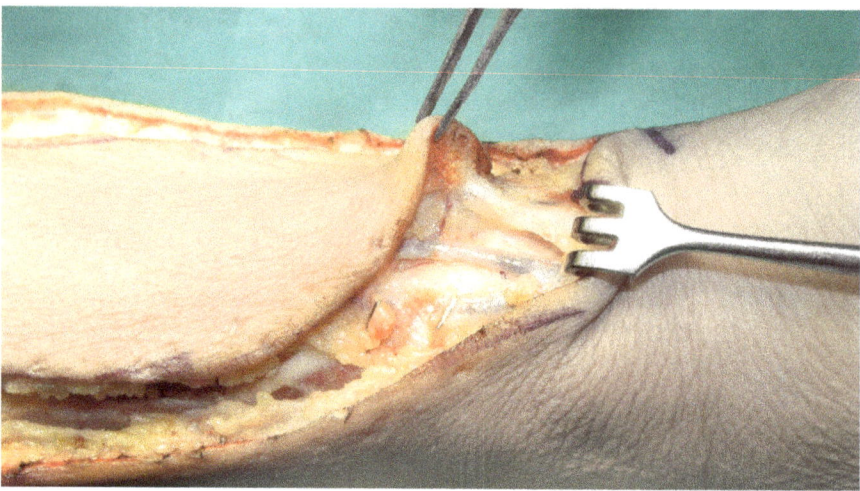

Fig. 18: There is constant tributary of cephalic vein over radial artery.

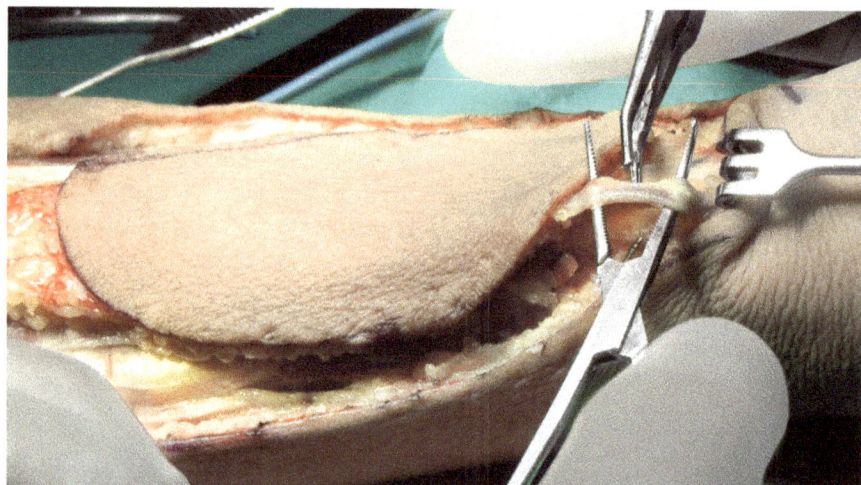

Fig. 19: Vein is ligated with ligaclips.

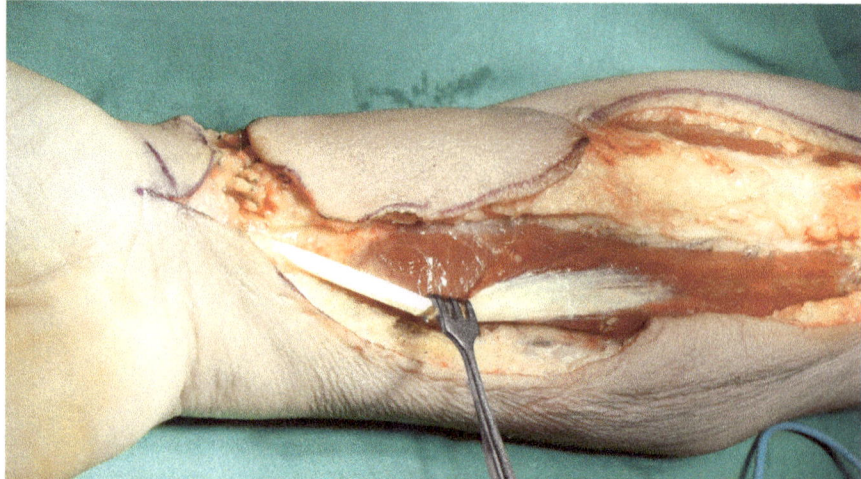

Fig. 20: Flap is raised from distal to proximal in subfascial plane between flexor carpi radialis and brachioradialis.

Operative Steps of Free Radial Artery Forearm Flap

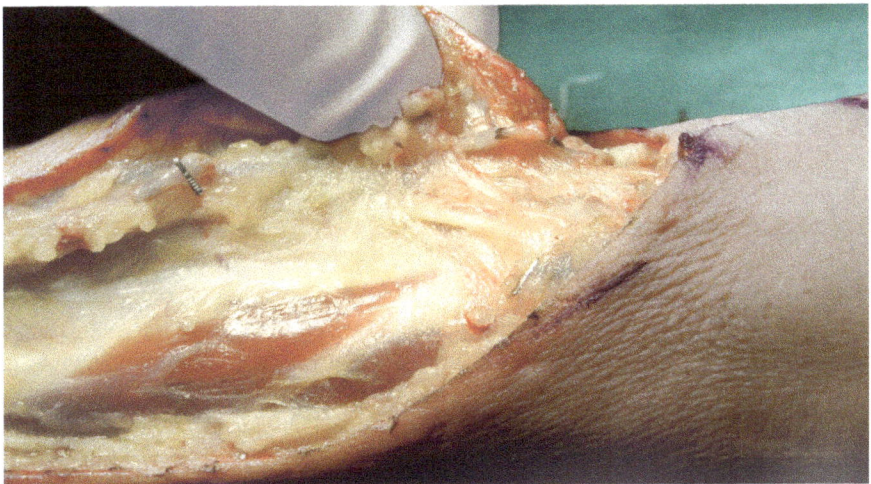

Fig. 21: We preserved one of the three branches of radial sensory nerve.

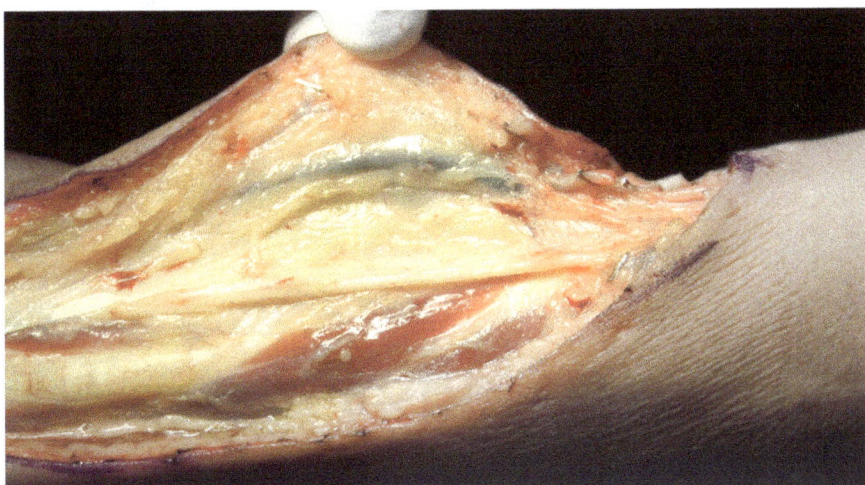

Fig. 22: Pedicle and sensory radial nerve is seen.

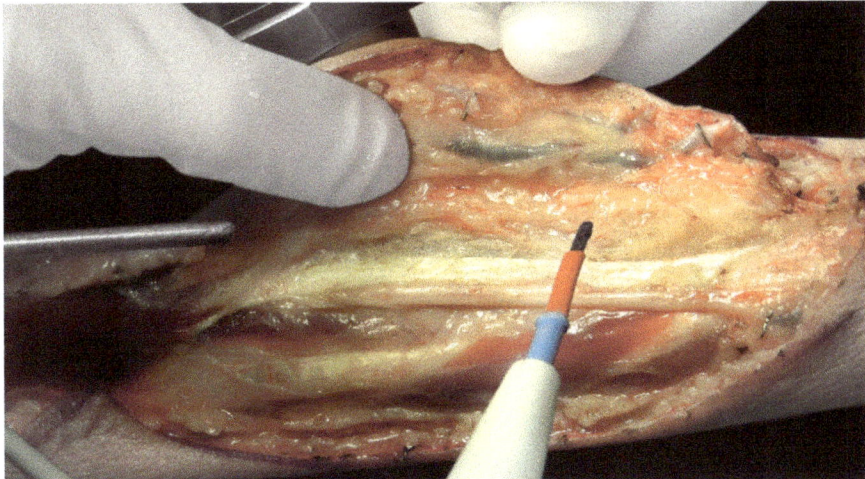

Fig. 23: Subfascial dissection of flap medial to brachioradialis is seen.

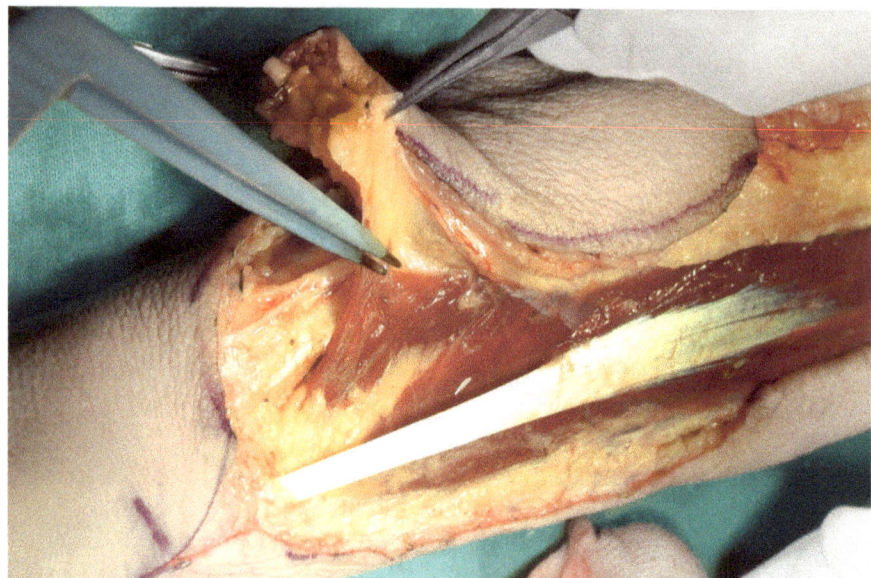

Fig. 24: A pad of fat is dissected with bipolar cautery from distal to proximal.

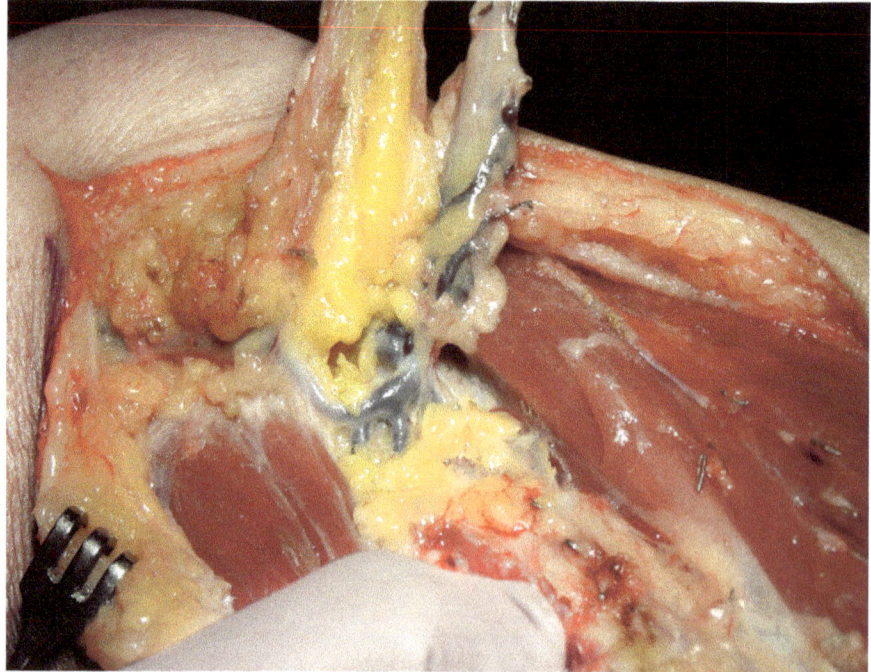

Fig. 25: Venae comitantes[8] are draining in medial cubital vein at elbow.

Operative Steps of Free Radial Artery Forearm Flap

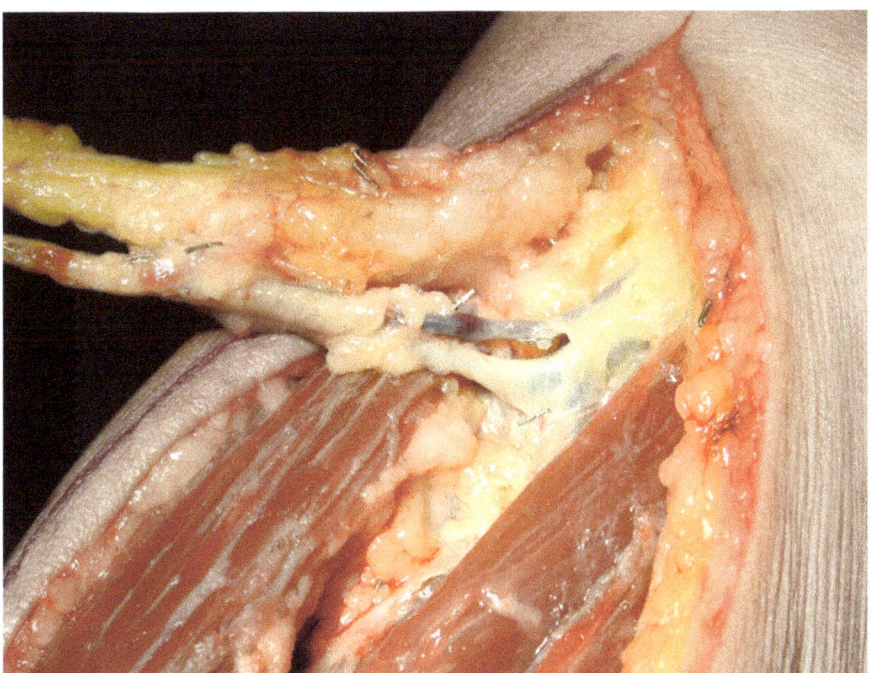

Fig. 26: Dissection is completed at elbow.

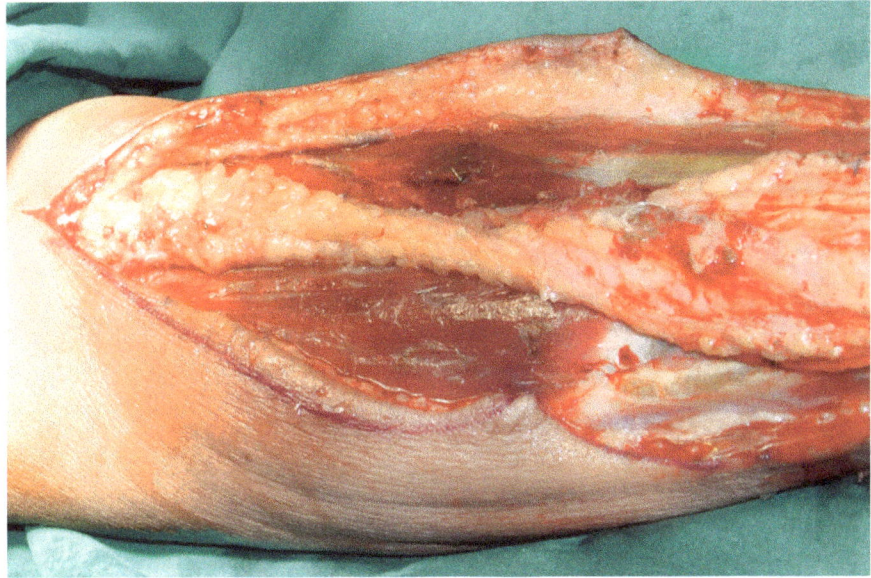

Fig. 27: Tourniquet is released and hemostasis is done.

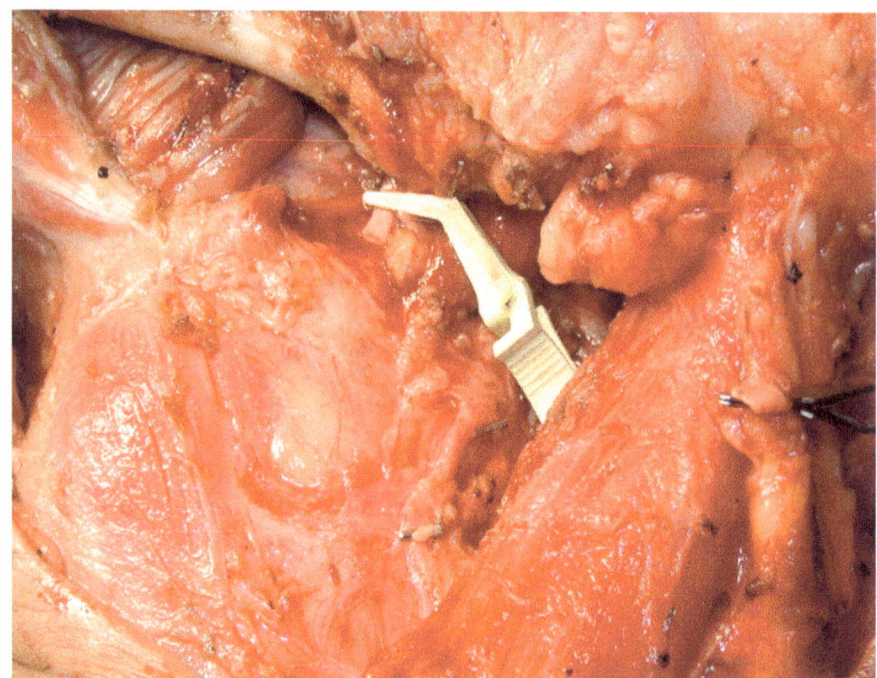

Fig. 28: Clamps are applied over facial artery and external jugular vein.

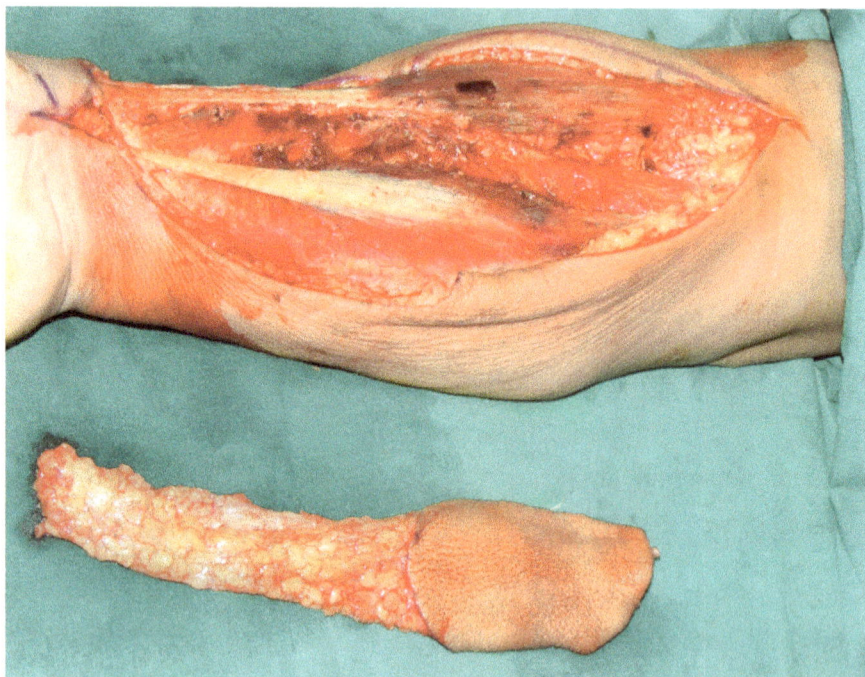

Fig. 29: Flap is divided.

Operative Steps of Free Radial Artery Forearm Flap

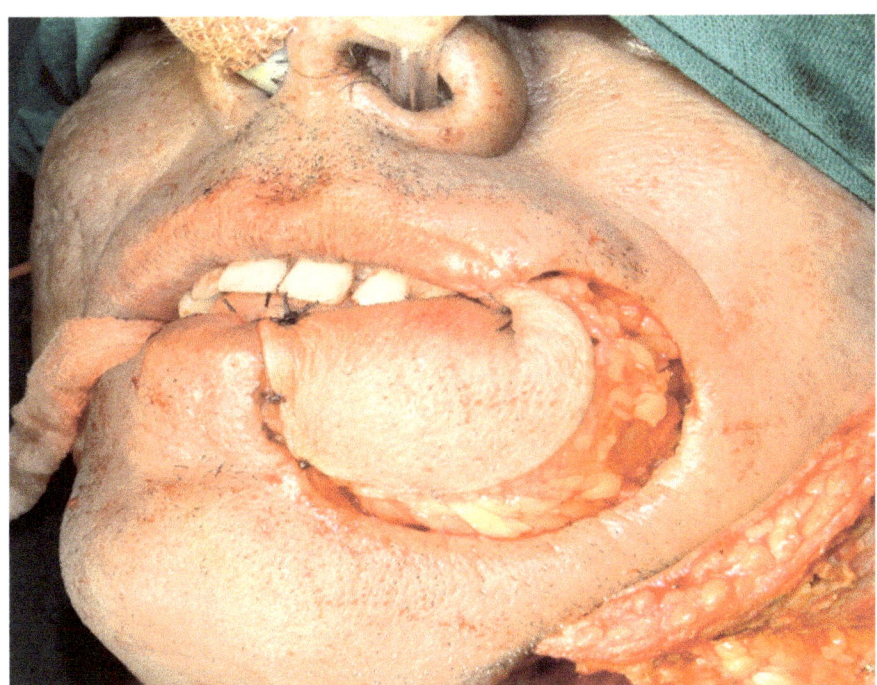

Fig. 30: Inset is given for inner lining first.

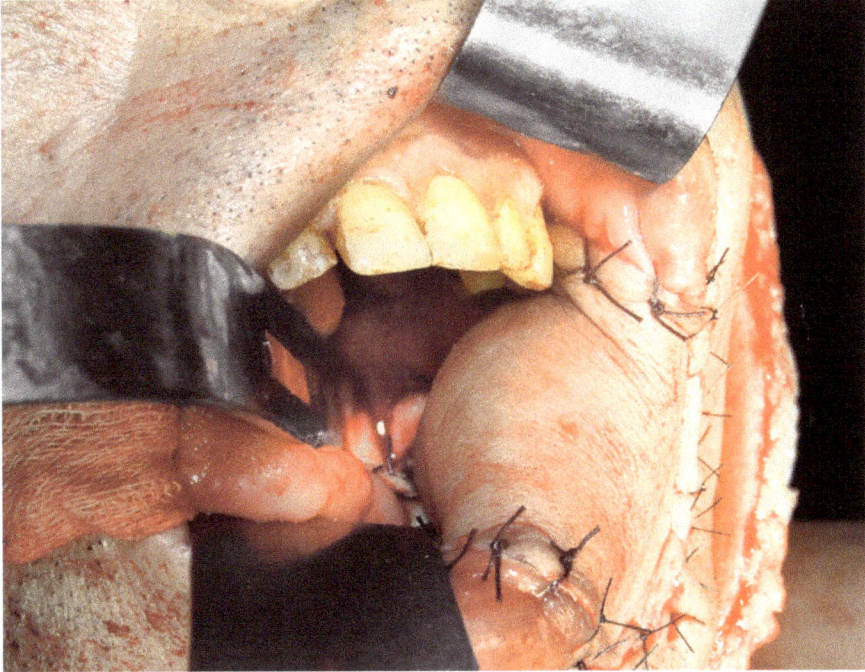

Fig. 31: Inset is completed.

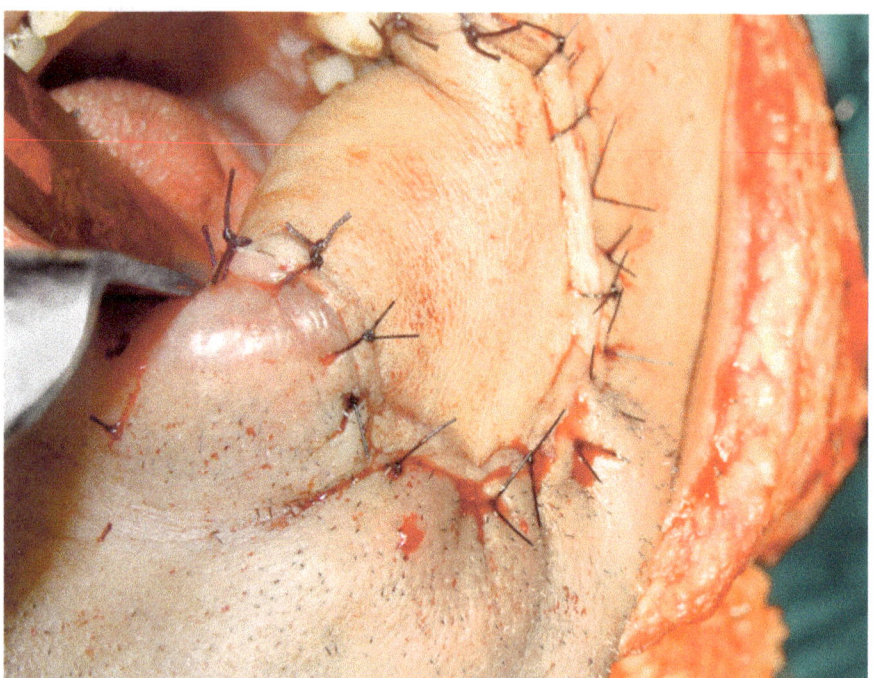

Fig. 32: Free radial artery forearm flap gives better cosmetic result.

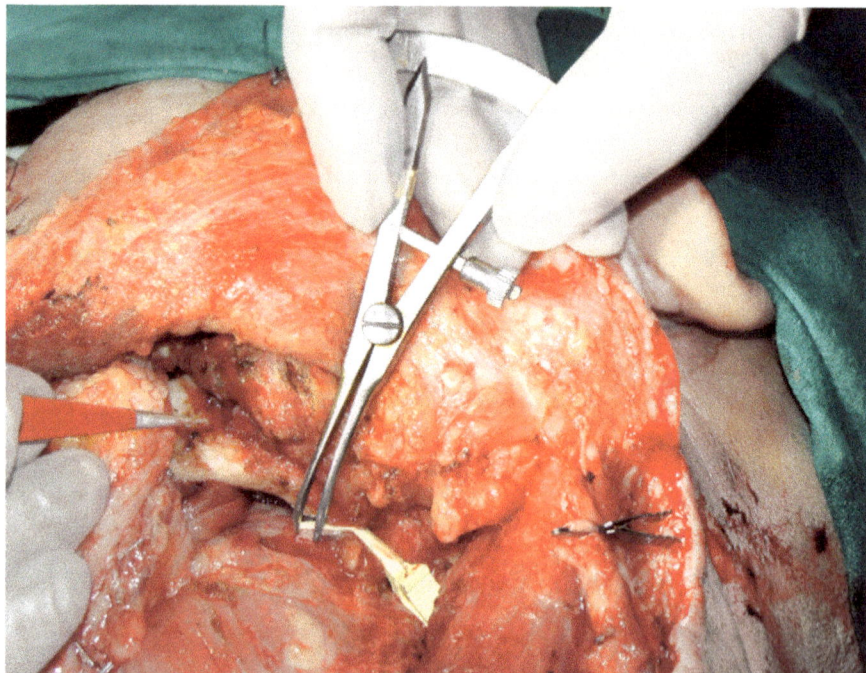

Fig. 33: Facial artery has 3.2 mm diameter.

Operative Steps of Free Radial Artery Forearm Flap

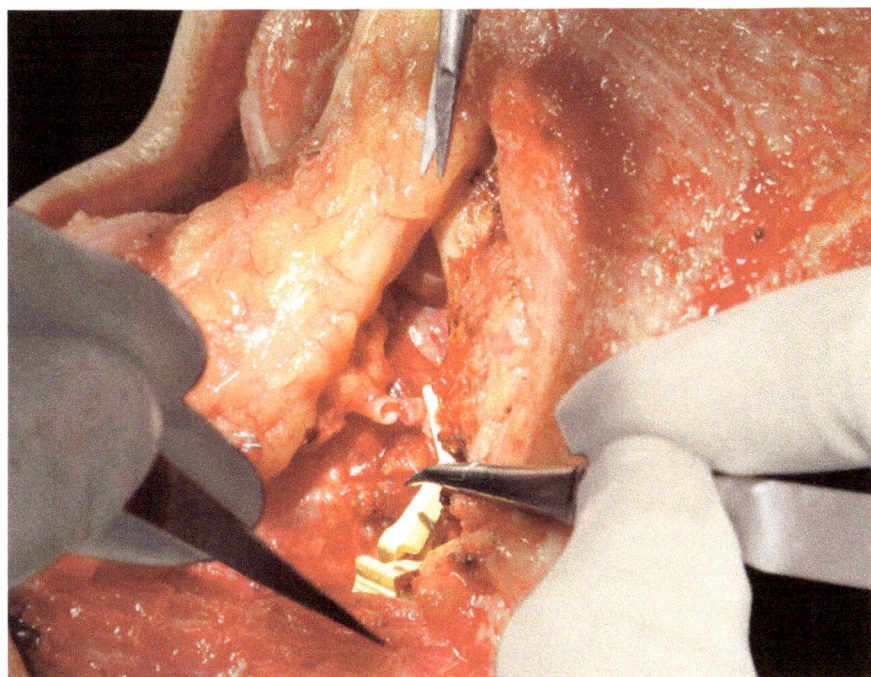

Fig. 34: Facial artery is sutured to radial artery with 8-0 prolene.

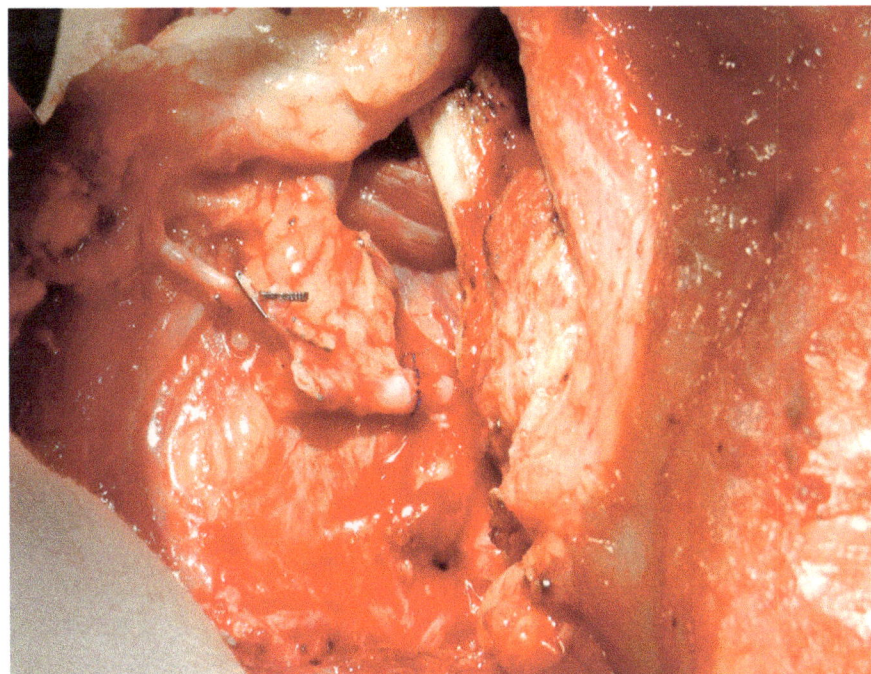

Fig. 35: Arterial anastomosis is completed.

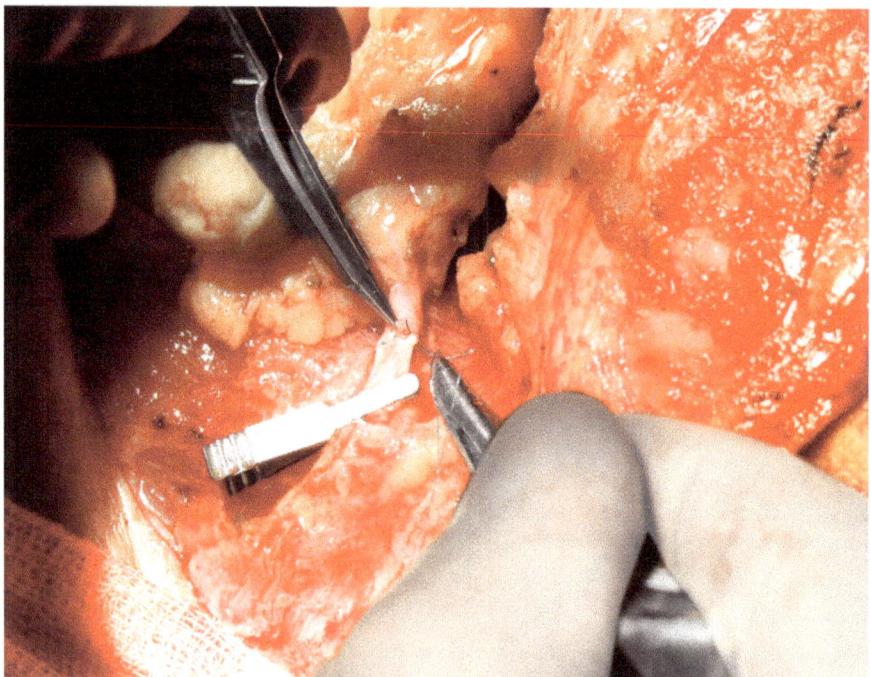

Fig. 36: Cephalic vein is anastomosed to external jugular vein with 8-0 prolene.

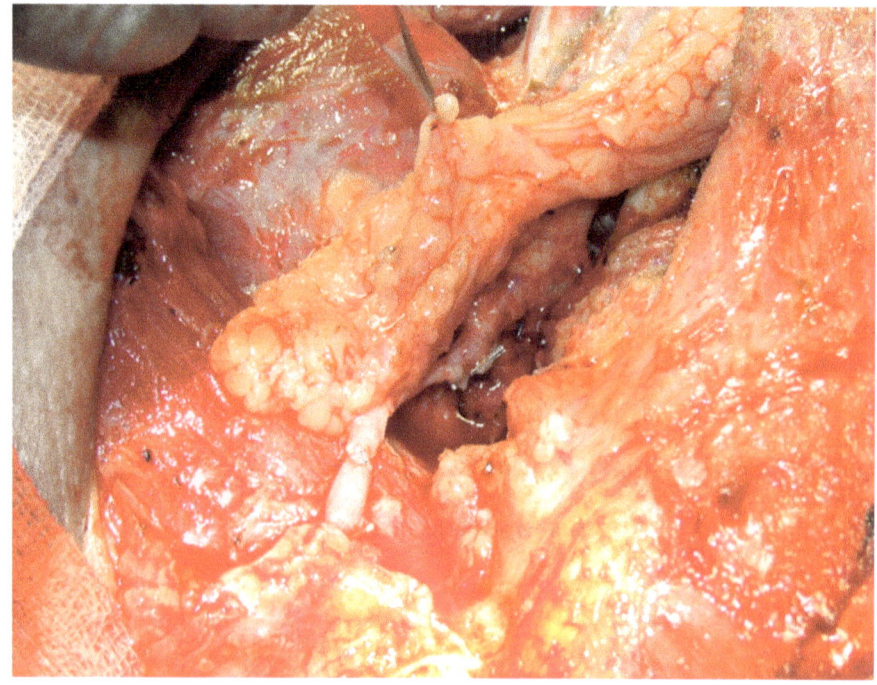

Fig. 37: Venous anastomosis completed.

Operative Steps of Free Radial Artery Forearm Flap

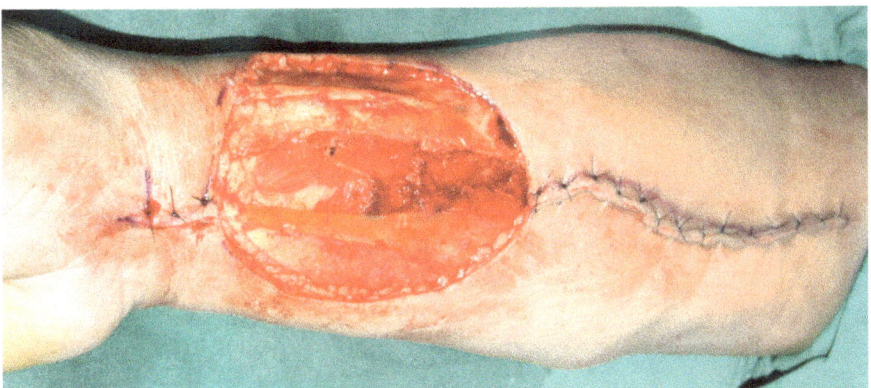
Fig. 38: Incision is sutured with 3-0 ethilon.

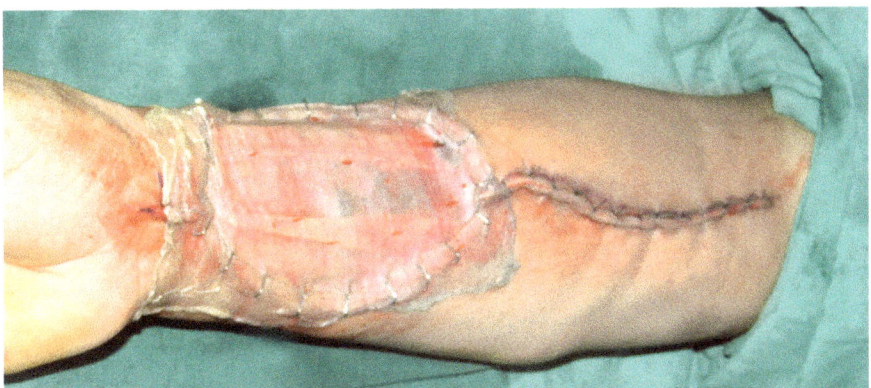
Fig. 39: Split thickness skin graft is taken from thigh and placed over donor site of flap.

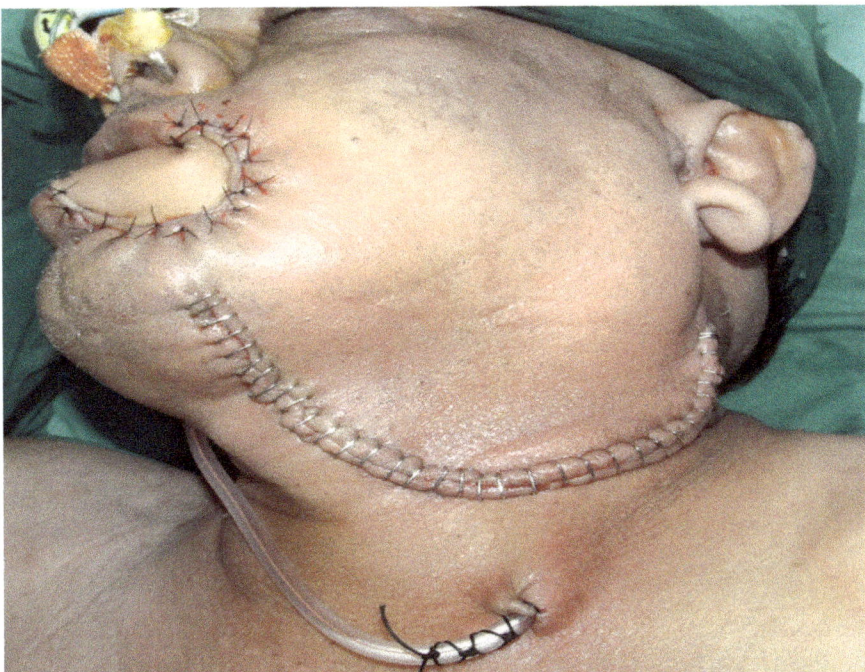
Fig. 40: Drain is kept away from anastomosis sites and wound is closed layerwise.

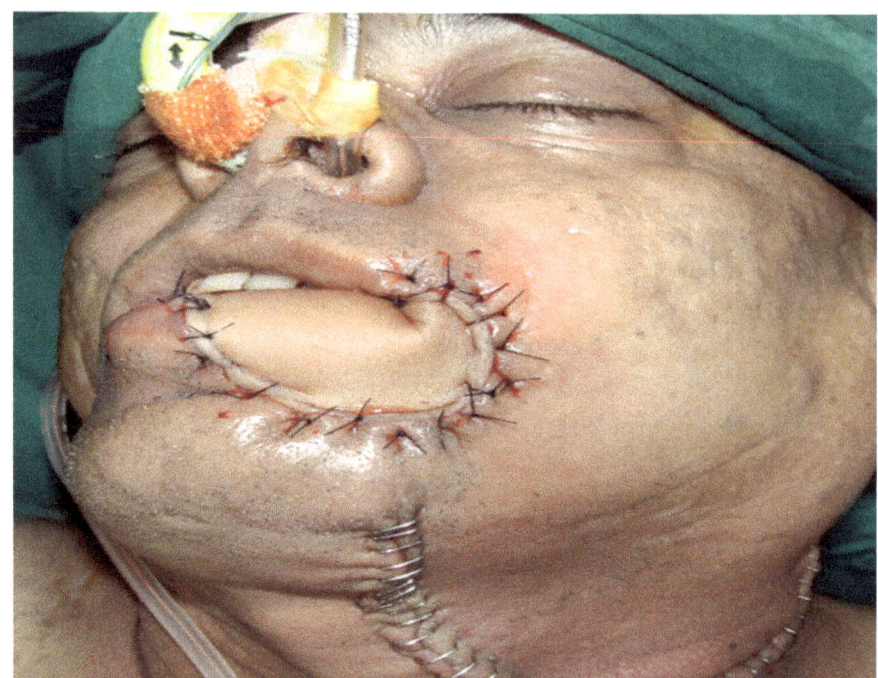

Fig. 41: Suturing completed.

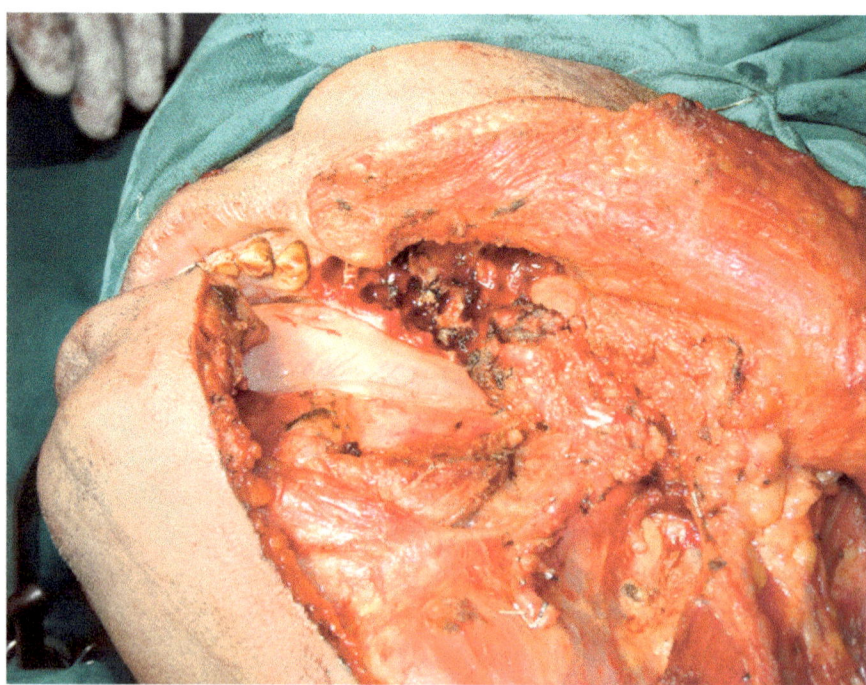

Fig. 42: Modified neck dissection and excision of carcinoma buccal mucosa is done.

Operative Steps of Free Radial Artery Forearm Flap

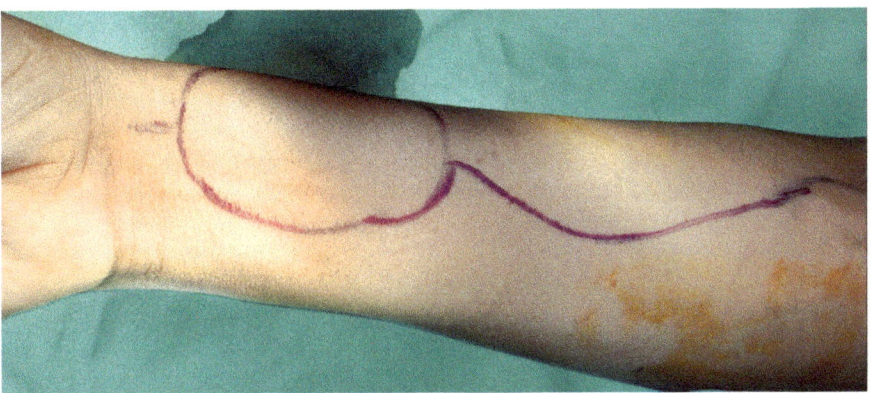

Fig. 43: Marking is done.

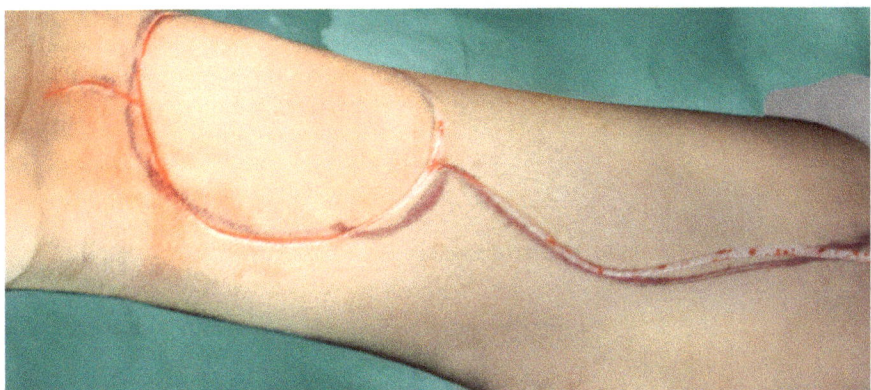

Fig. 44: Incision is kept.

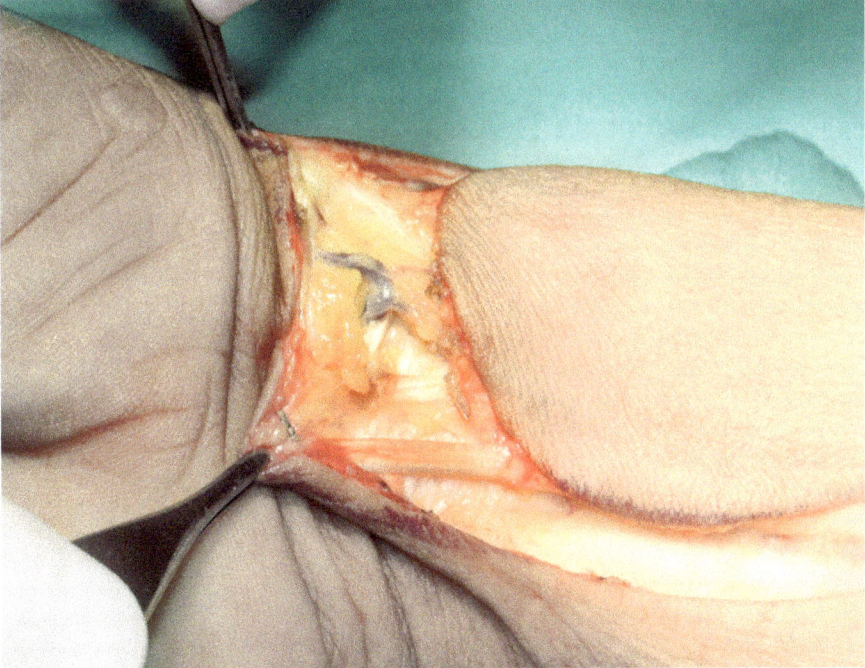

Fig. 45: Vein is ligated.

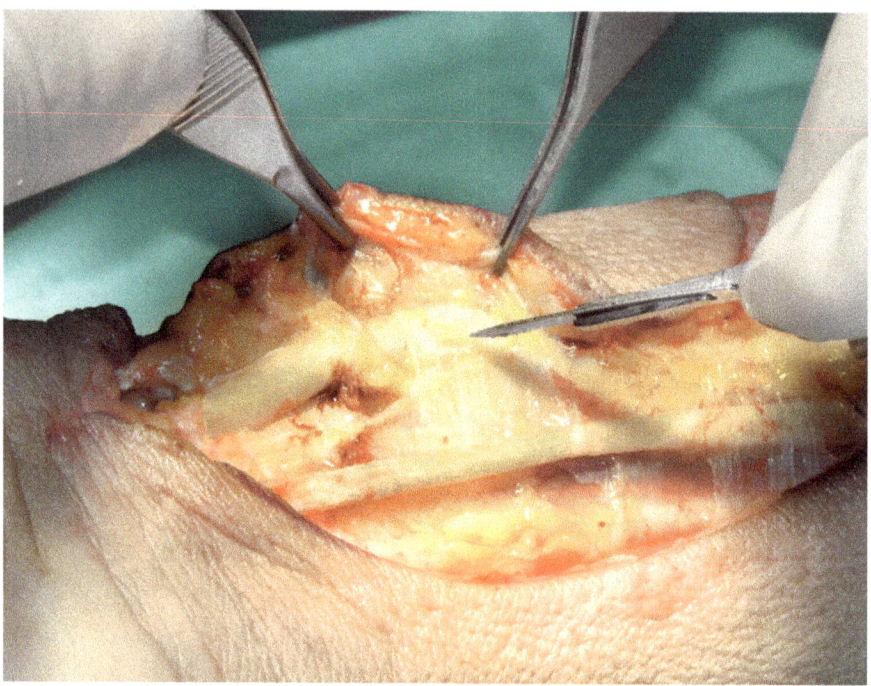

Fig. 46: Flap dissection on ulnar aspect.

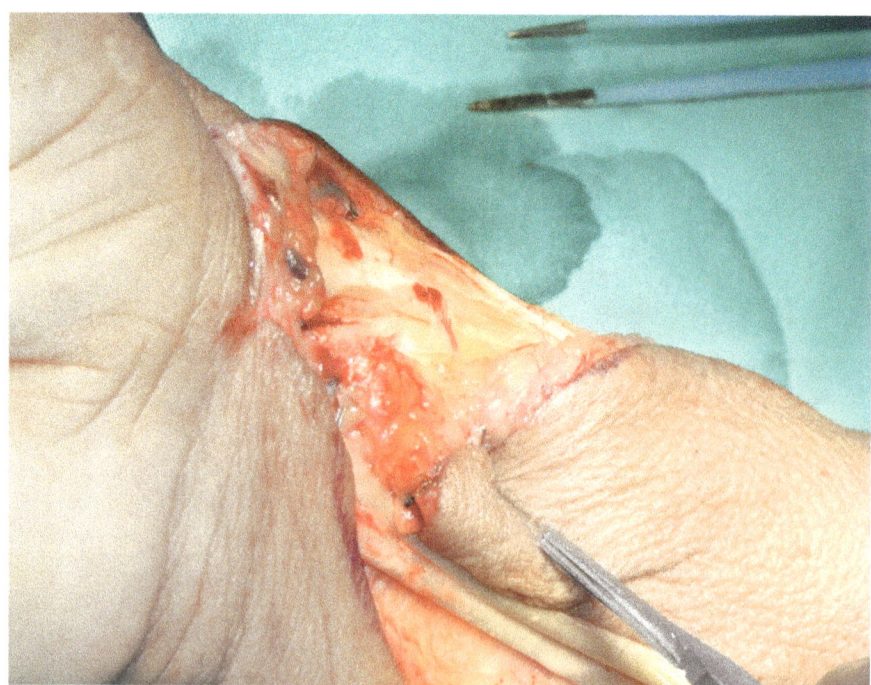

Fig. 47: Flap is dissected from distal to proximal in subfascial plane between flexor carpi radialis and brachioradialis.

Operative Steps of Free Radial Artery Forearm Flap

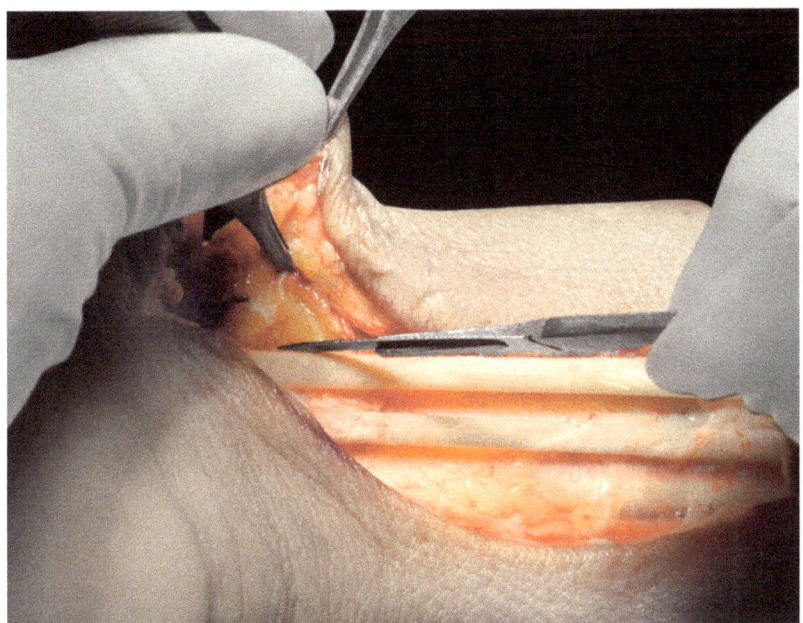

Fig. 48: Dissection is carried out in subfascial plane at radial border of flexor carpi radialis.

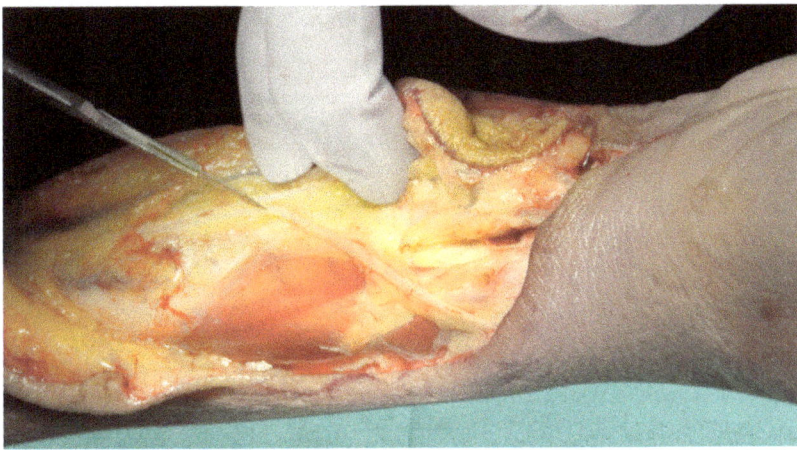

Fig. 49: Sensory branch of radial nerve is saved.

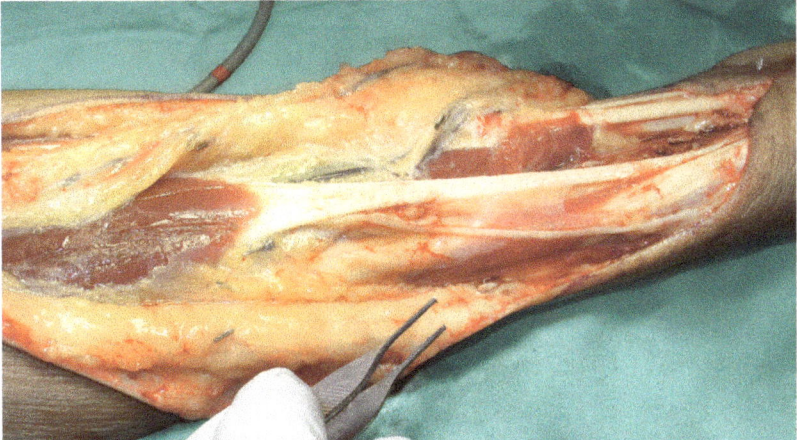

Fig. 50: Pedicle is close to brachioradialis and we have to be very careful while dissecting.

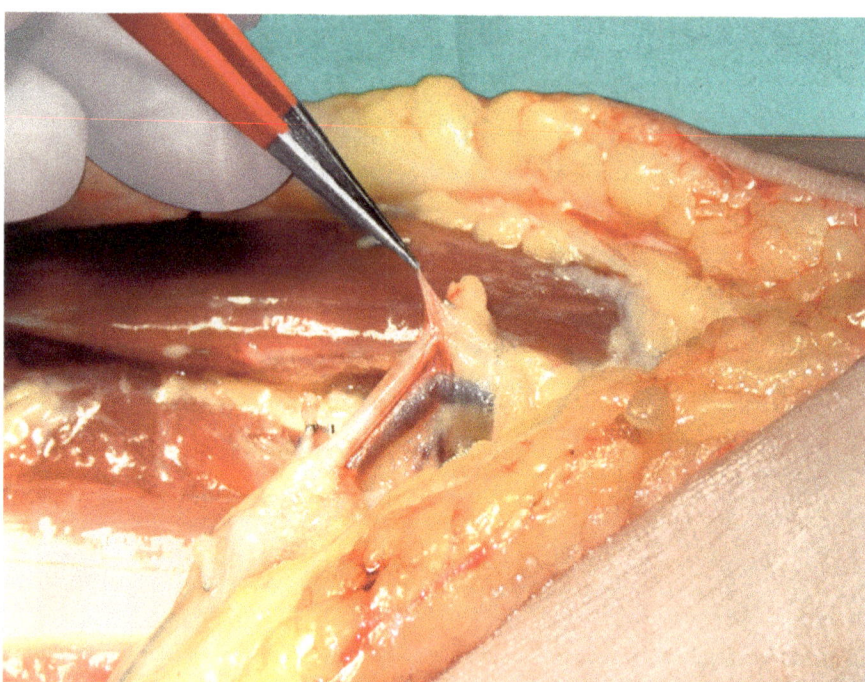
Fig. 51: Pedicle is seen at elbow.

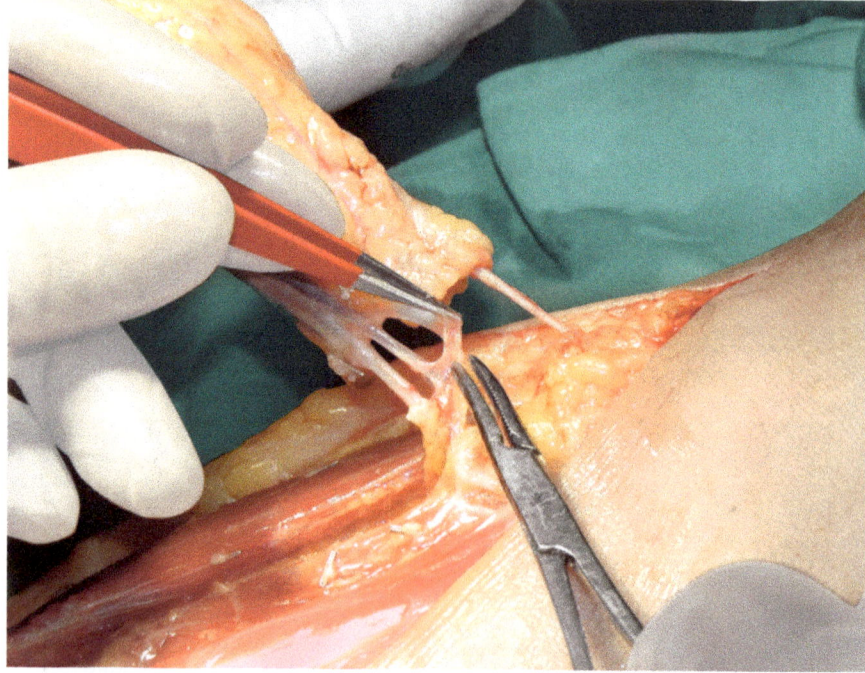
Fig. 52: Dissection of pedicle at elbow.

Operative Steps of Free Radial Artery Forearm Flap

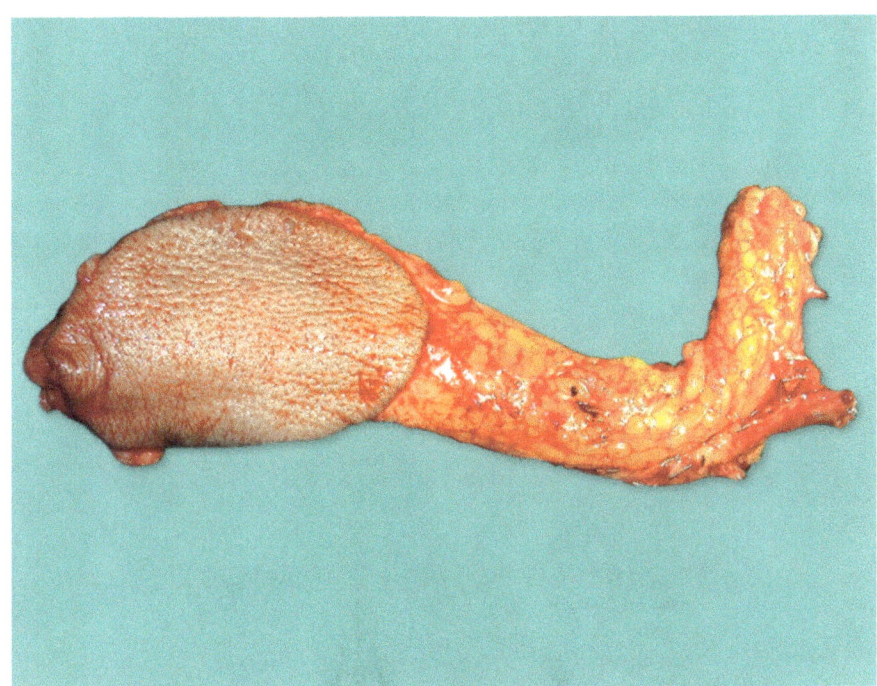

Fig. 53: Flap is divided.

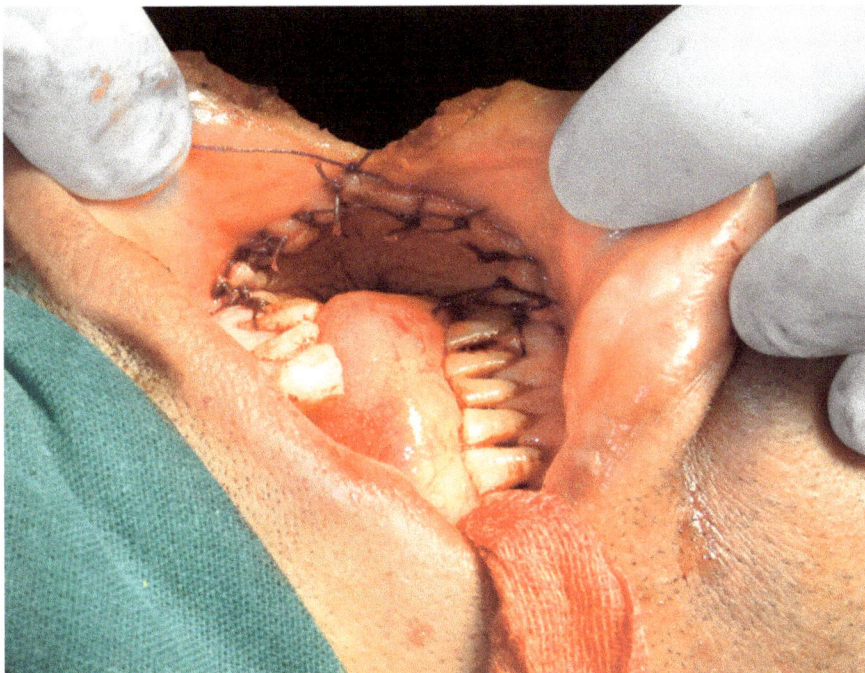

Fig. 54: Inset is done with 2-0 vicryl.

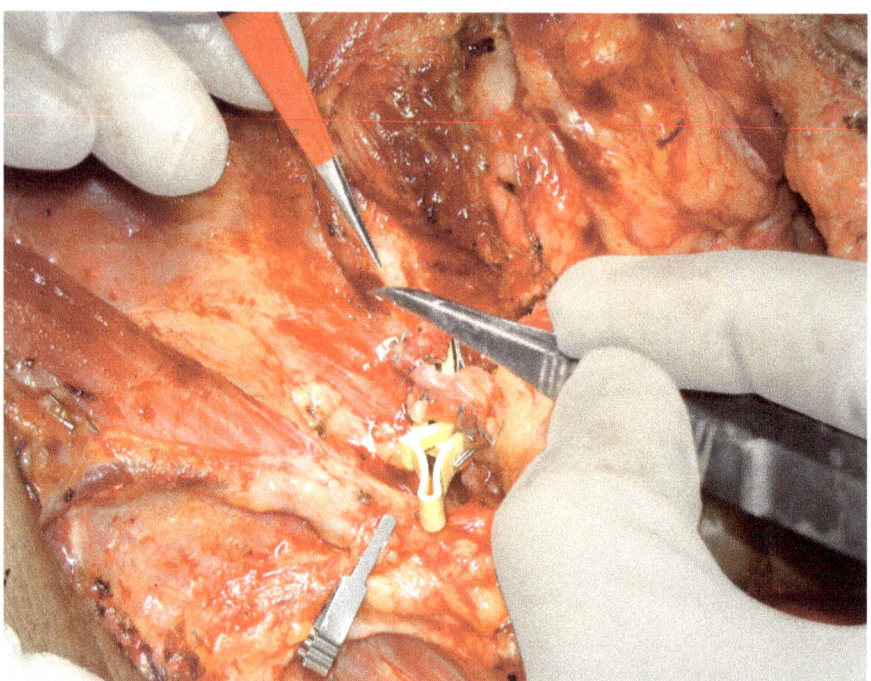

Fig. 55: Facial artery anastomosed to radial artery.

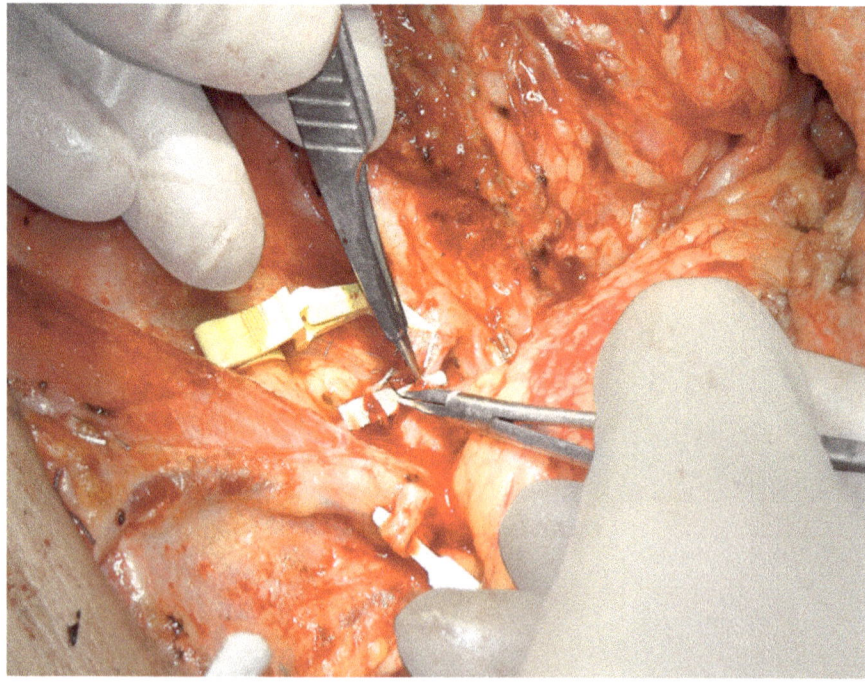

Fig. 56: Venae comitant is sutured to facial vein with 10-0 ethilon.

Operative Steps of Free Radial Artery Forearm Flap

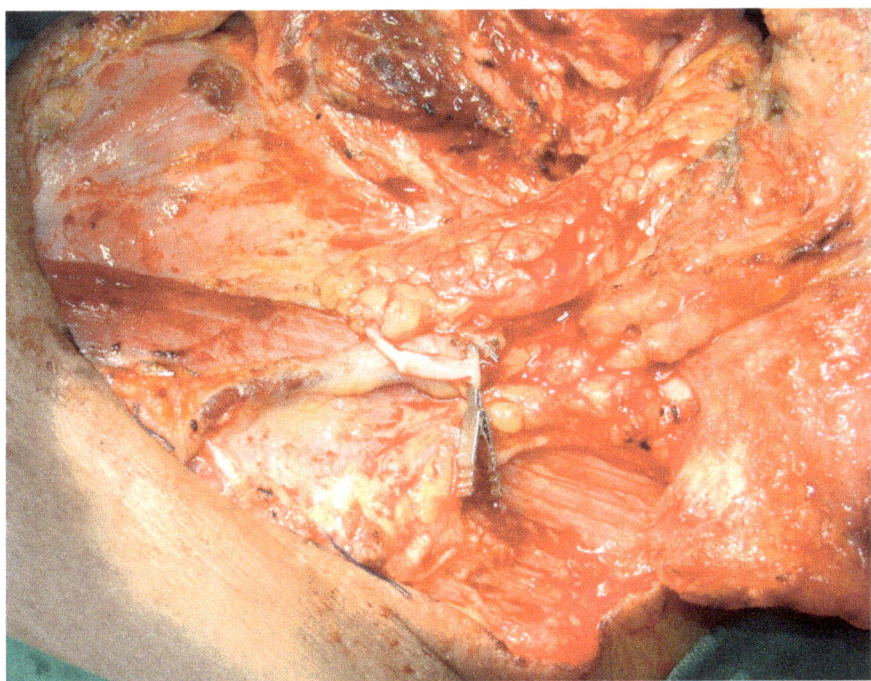

Fig. 57: Cephalic vein is anastomosed to external jugular vein.

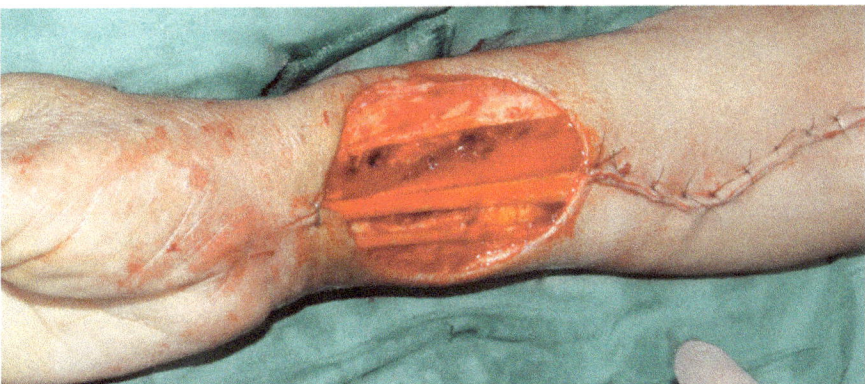

Fig. 58: Donor site.

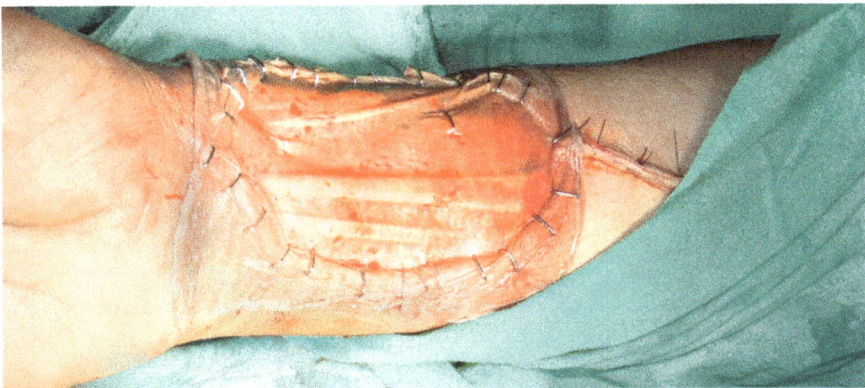

Fig. 59: Split thickness skin graft placed over donor site of flap.

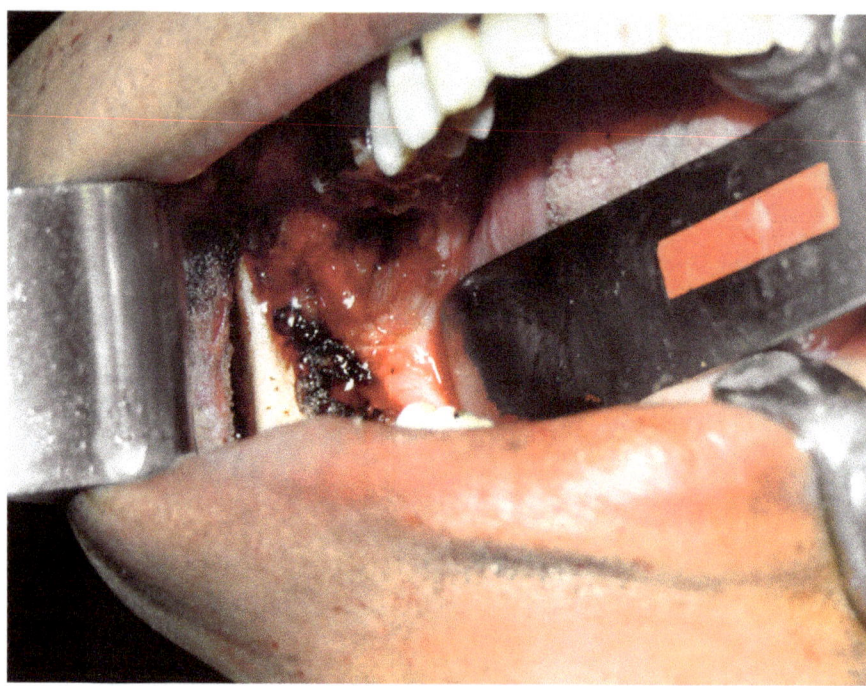

Fig. 60: Intraoral excision of carcinoma buccal mucosa done.

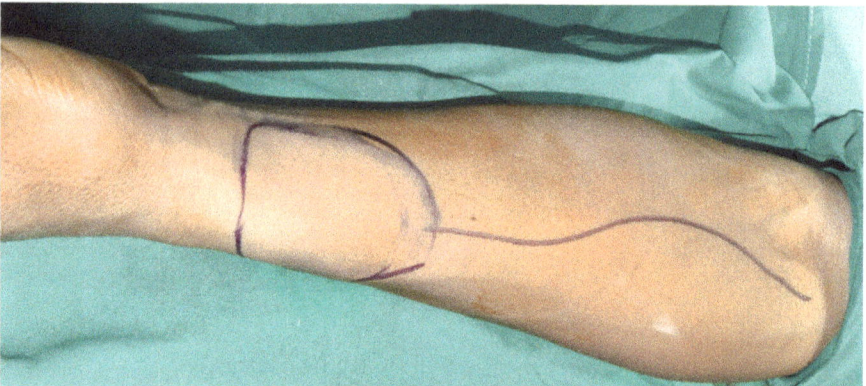

Fig. 61: Marking is done.

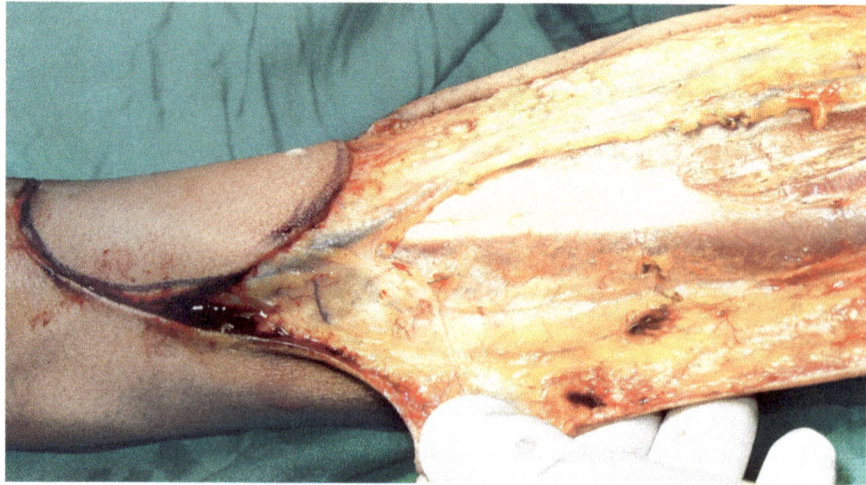

Fig. 62: Cephalic vein is dissected.

Operative Steps of Free Radial Artery Forearm Flap

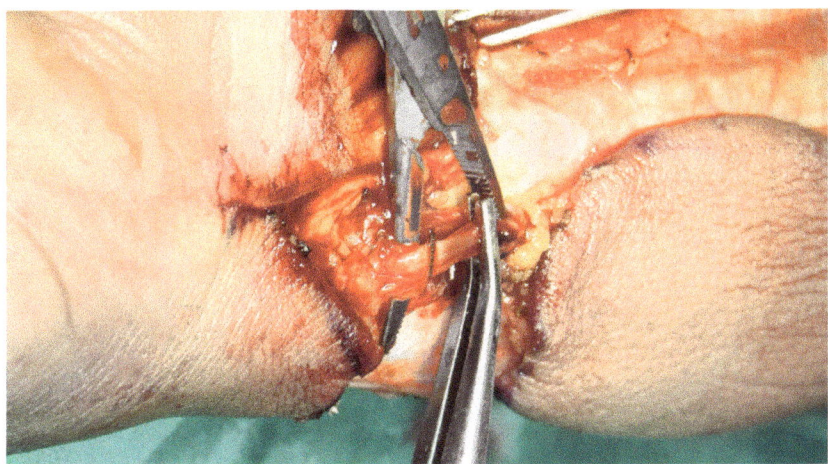

Fig. 63: Distally radial artery is ligated and cut.

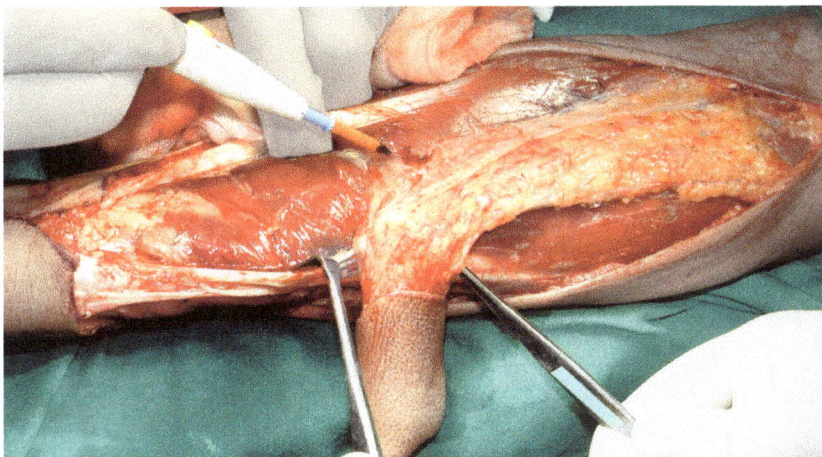

Fig. 64: Flap is dissected.

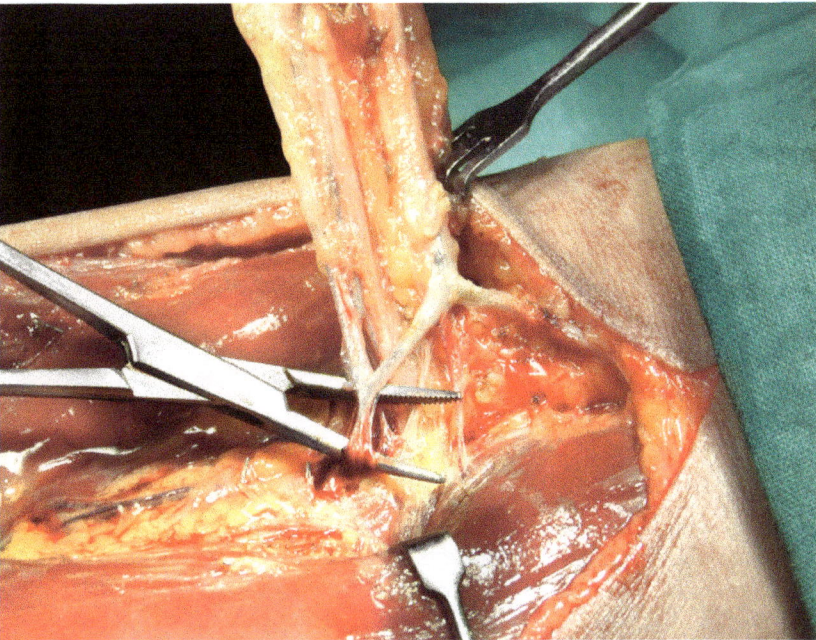

Fig. 65: Venae comitant is draining in medial cubital vein.

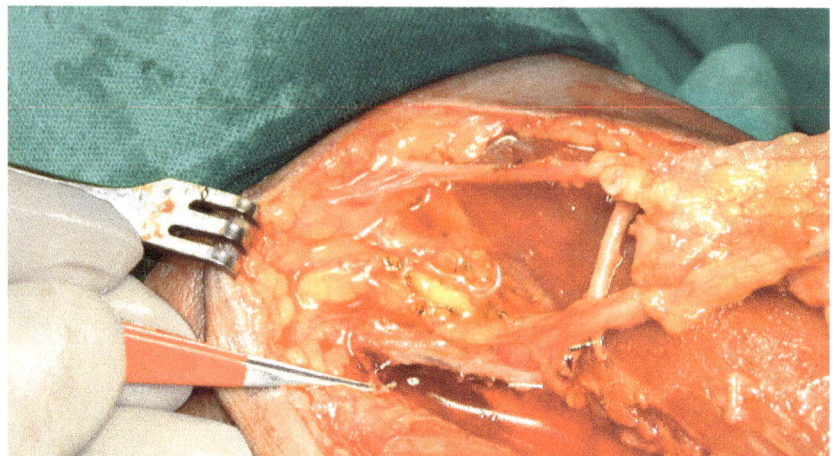

Fig. 66: Vessels at elbow.

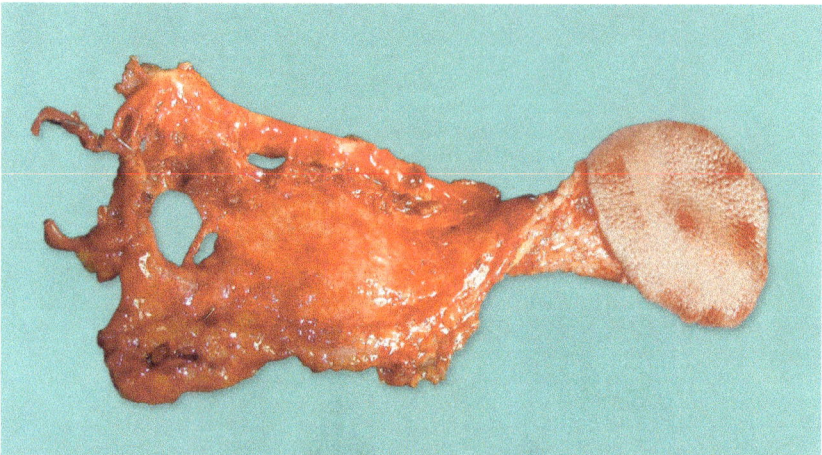

Fig. 67: Flap is divided.

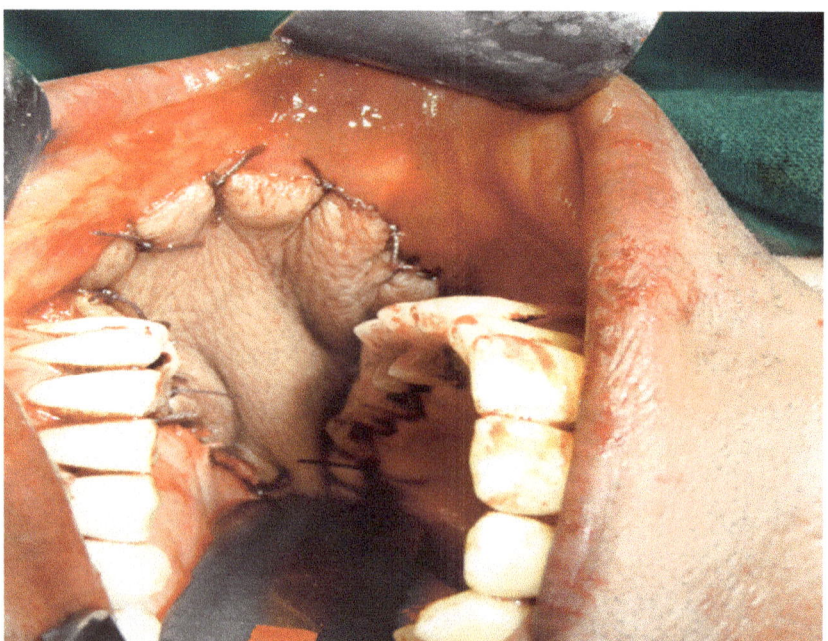

Fig. 68: Inset is given with 2-0 vicryl.

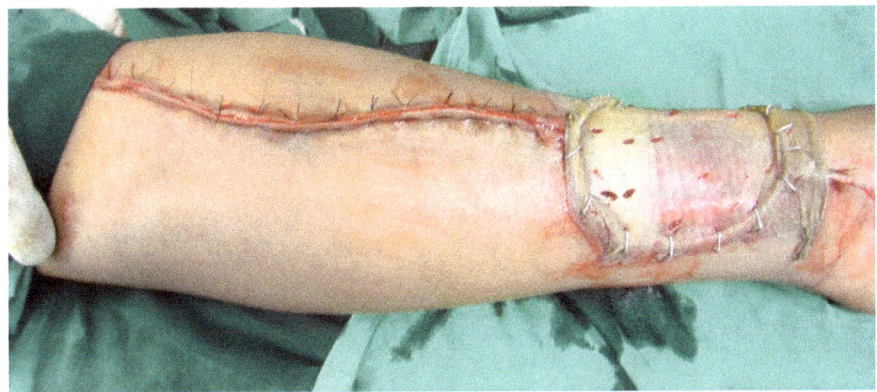

Fig. 69: Split thickness skin graft taken from thigh and placed over donor site of flap.[9]

REFERENCES

1. Harashina T, Fujino T, Aoyagi F. Reconstruction of the oral cavity with a free flap. Plast Reconstr Surg. 1976:58:412-4.
2. Panje WR, Bardach J, Krause CJ. Reconstruction of the oral cavity with a free flap. Plast Reconstr Surg. 1976:58:415-8.
3. Evans HB, Lampe HB. The radial artery forearm flap in head and neck reconstruction. J Otolaryngol. 1987:16:382-6.
4. Chang SC, Miller G, Halbert CF, Cher TS, Chen IH. Limiting donor site morbidity by suprafascial dissection of the radial artery forearm flap. Microsurgery. 1996;17;136-40.
5. Brenner P, Berger A, Caspary L. Angiologic observations following autologous vein grafting and free radial artery flap elevation. J Reconstr Microsurg. 1988;4:297-301.
6. Jones BM, O'Brien CJ. Acute ischaemia of the hand resulting from elevation of a radial forearm flap. Br J Plast Surg. 1985;38:396-7.
7. Meland NB, Core GB, Hoverman VR. The radial forearm flap donor site: should we vein graft the artery? A comparative study. Plast Reconstr Surg. 1993;91:865-70.
8. Demirkan F, Wei FC, Lutz BS, Yang KH, Chao WC, Wei FC. Reliability of the venae comitantes in venous drainage of the free radial artery forearm flap. Plast Reconstr Surg. 1998;102:1544-8.
9. Swanson E, Boyd JB, Manktelow RT. The radial forearm flap: reconstructive applications and donor-site defects in 35 consecutive patients. Plast Reconstr Surg. 1990;85:258-66.

CHAPTER 7

Postoperative Care

All patients were kept in ICU for one day with awake intubation. Patients are extubated on next day morning.

THROMBOPROPHYLAXIS

Low molecular weight dextrose with 5000 units of heparin, 10 micro drops/minute is given for five days. The drops were reduced to 5 micro drops/minute, if there was bleeding from flap margin or sockets of teeth removed.

CHAPTER 8

Case Studies

CASE REPORTS

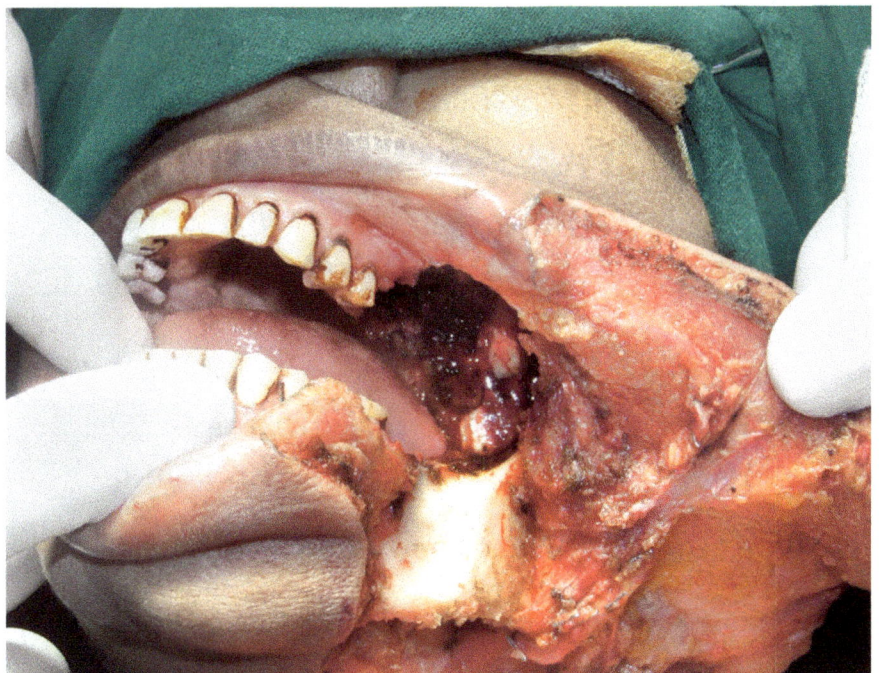

Fig. 1: Carcinoma of left buccal mucosa excision and upper alveolectomy is done.

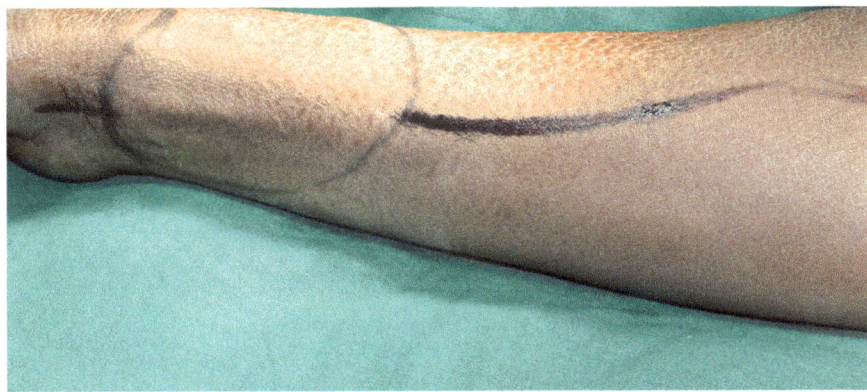

Fig. 2: Marking is done.

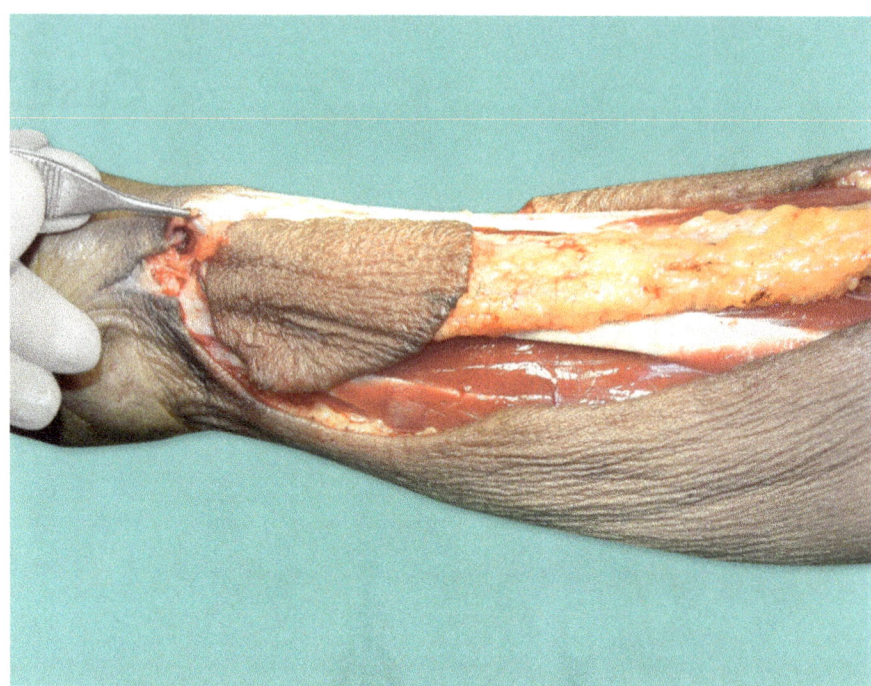

Fig. 3: Flap is dissected.

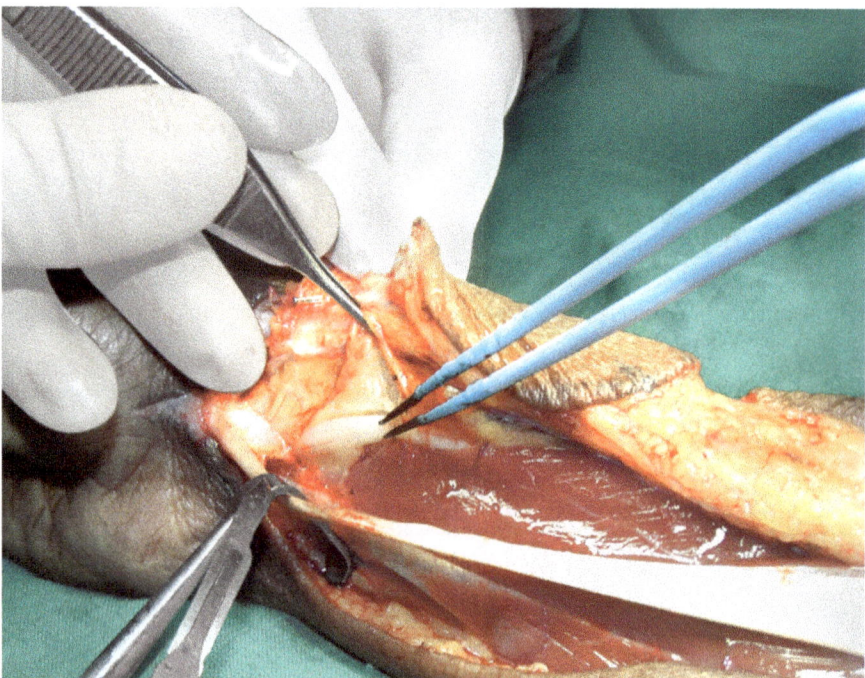

Fig. 4: Median nerve is seen.

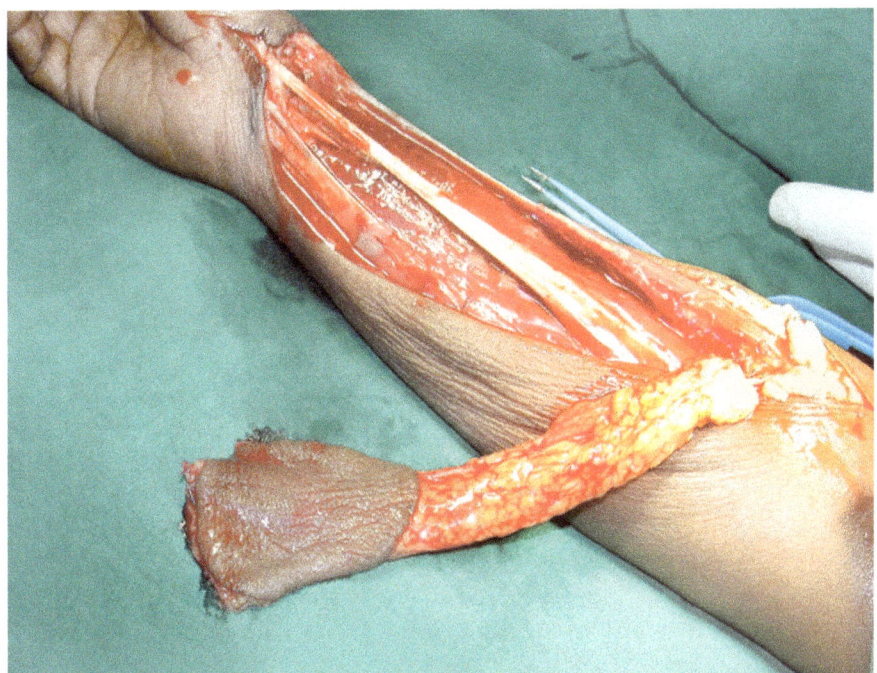

Fig. 5: Flap is harvested.

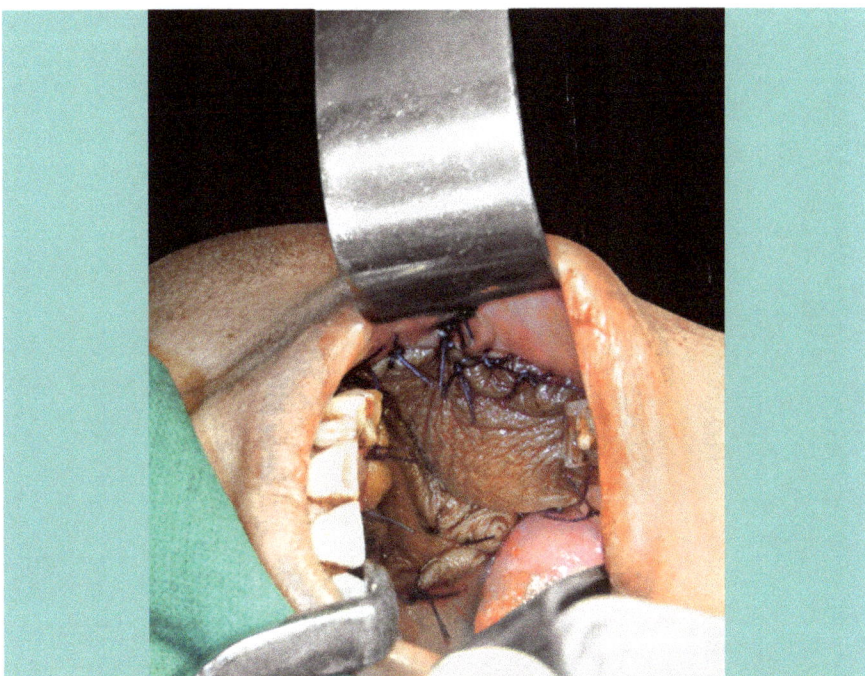

Fig. 6: Inset is given with 2-0 vicryl.

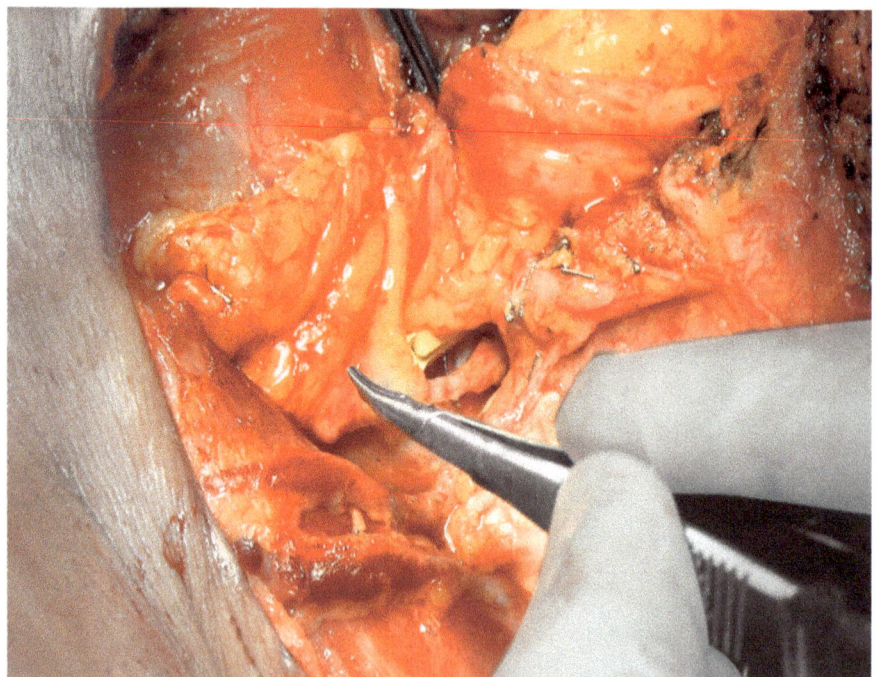

Fig. 7: Venae comitant is sutured with common facial vein with 10-0 ethilon.

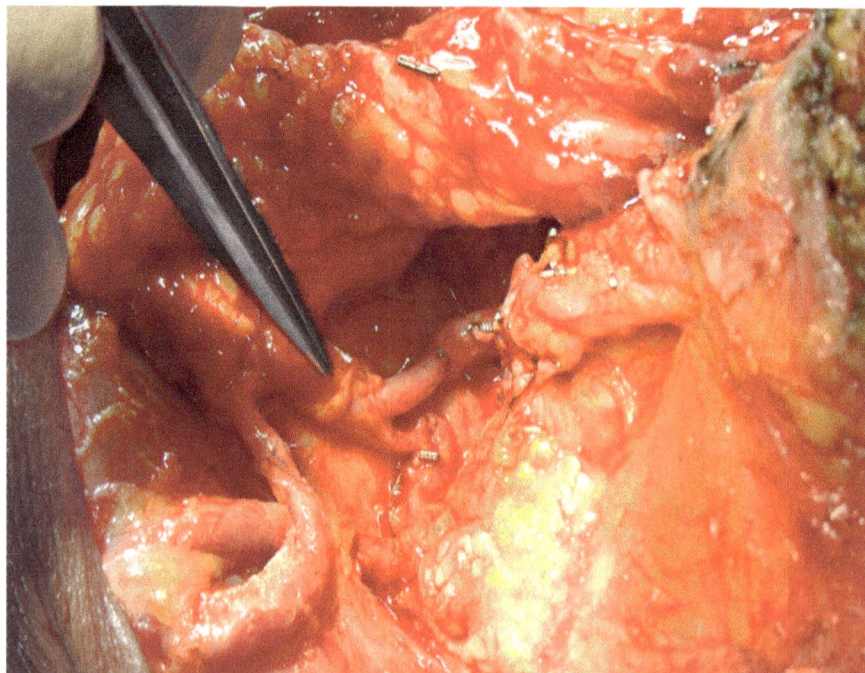

Fig. 8: Facial artery to radial artery, venae comitant to facial vein and cephalic vein to external jugular vein anastomosis were done.

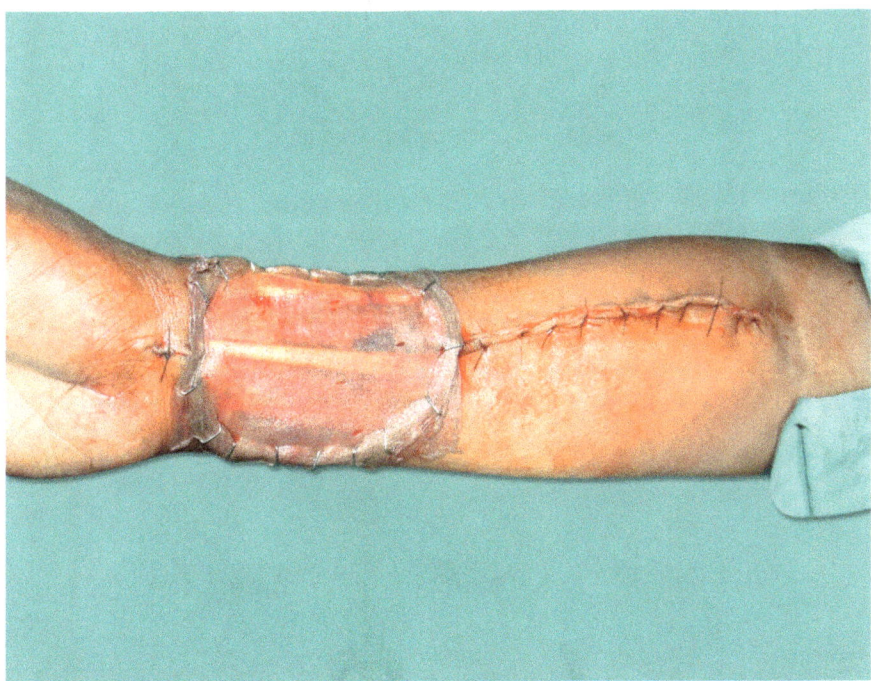

Fig. 9: Split thickness skin graft taken from thigh and placed over donor site of the flap.

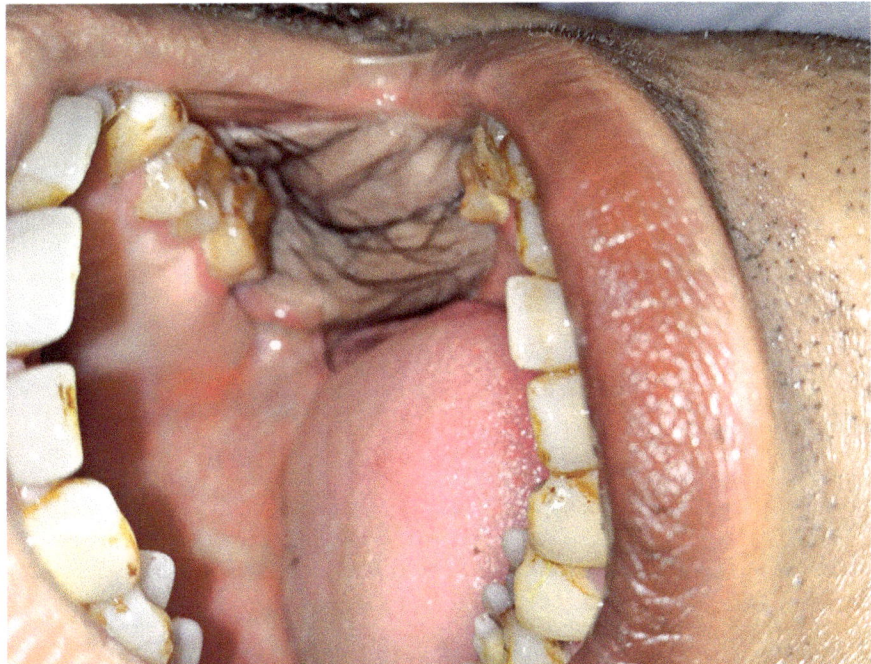

Fig. 10: Follow-up after one year.

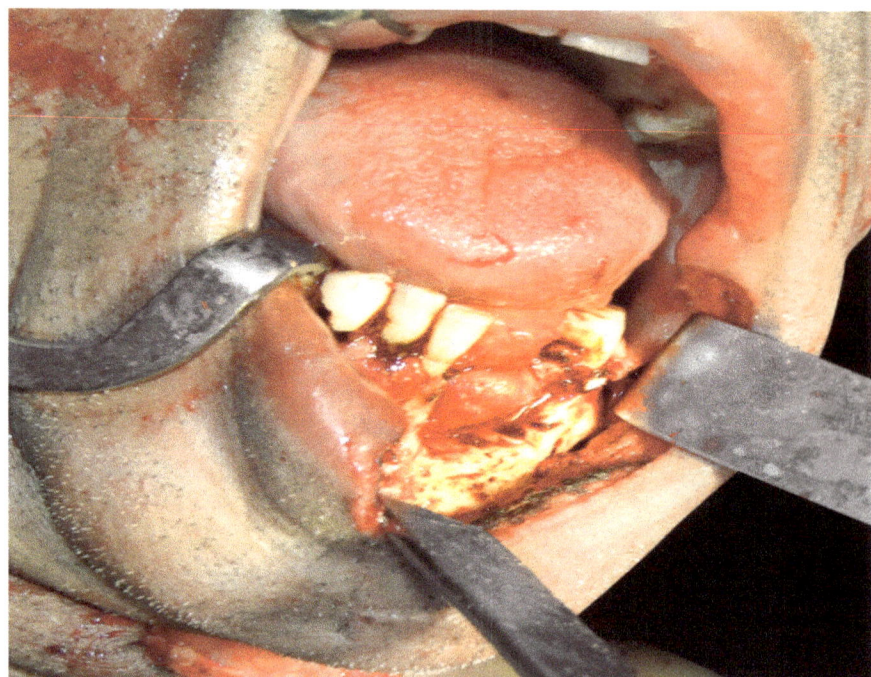

Fig. 11: Excision done of carcinoma of lower lip with marginal mandibulectomy.

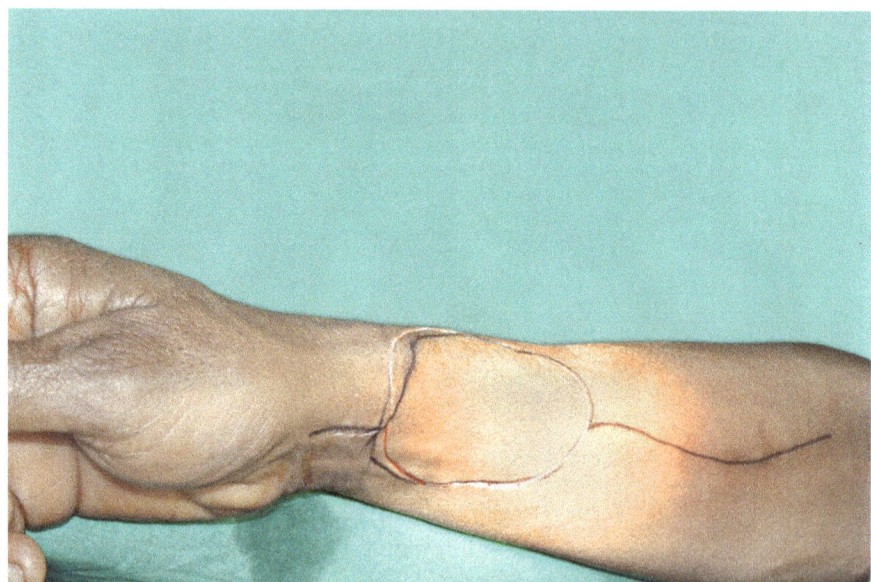

Fig. 12: Marking is done and incision is kept.

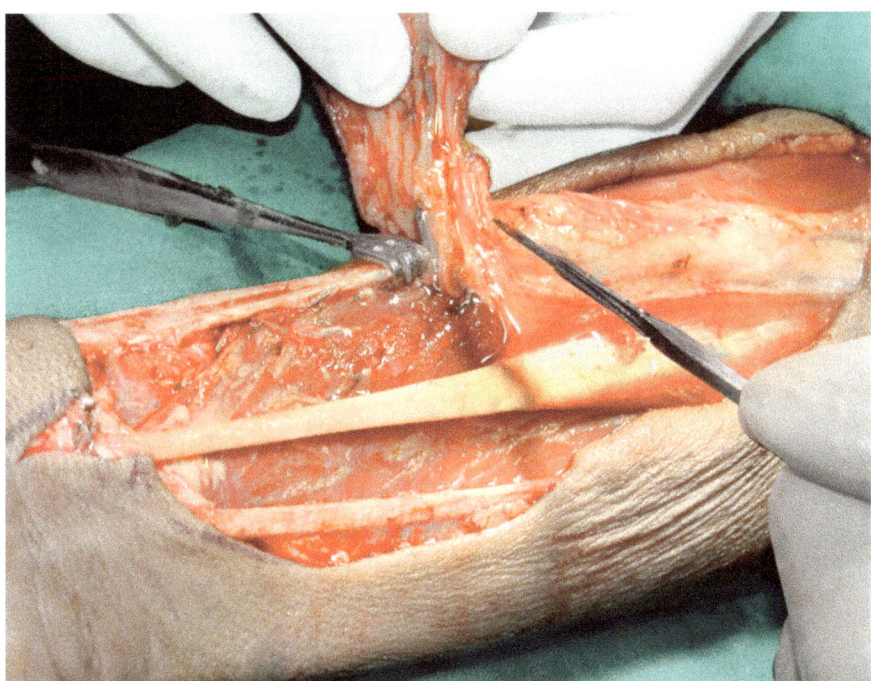

Fig. 13: Flap is raised.

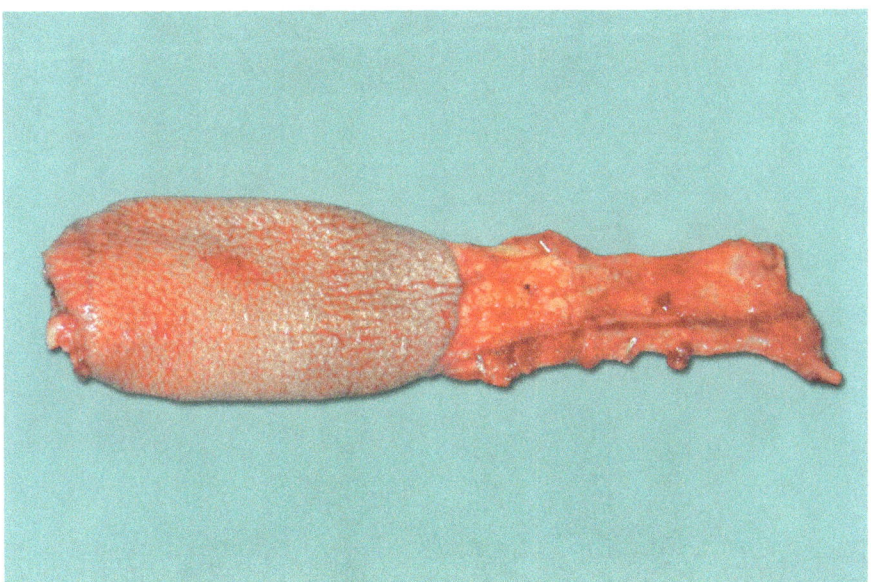

Fig. 14: Flap is harvested.

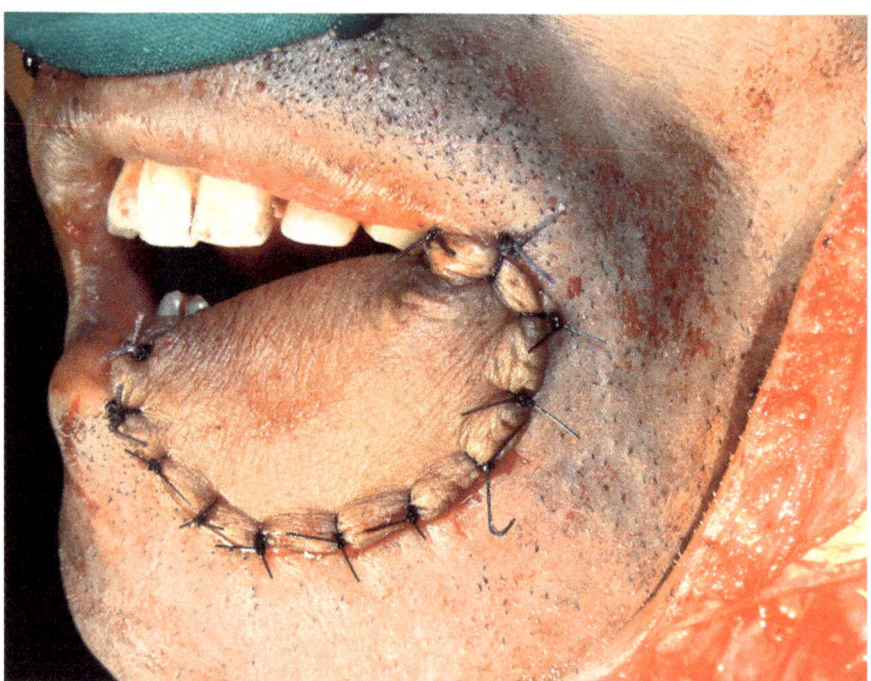

Fig. 15: Inset is completed.

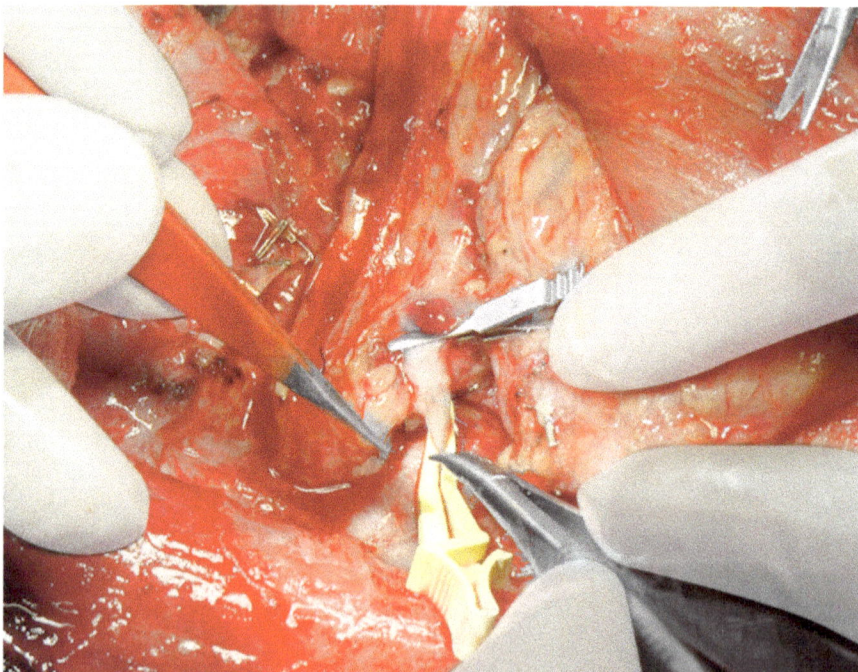

Fig. 16: Facial artery to radial artery, venae comitant to facial vein and cephalic vein to external jugular vein anastomosis were done.

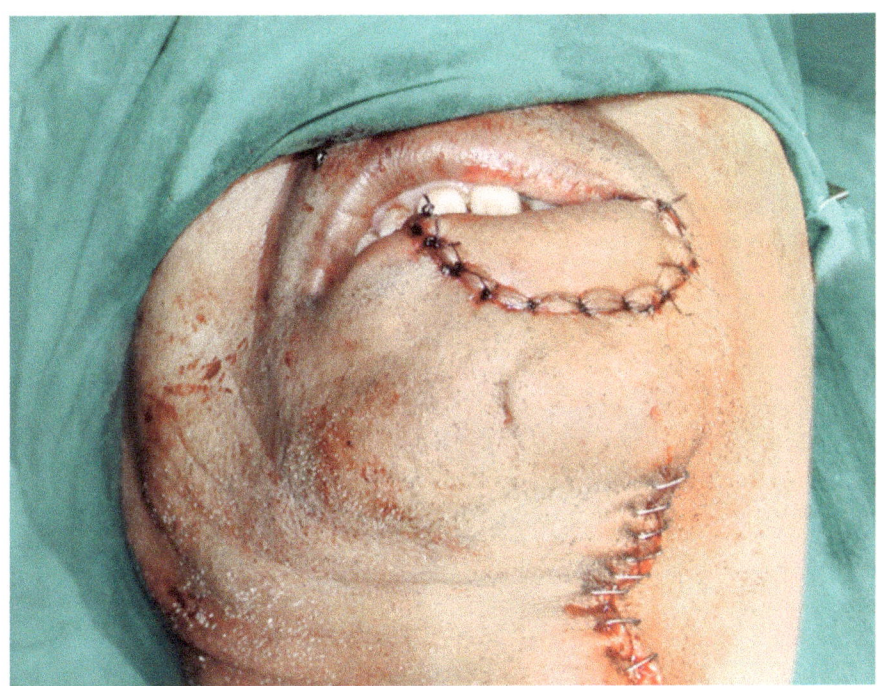

Fig. 17: After hemostasis neck was sutured layerwise.

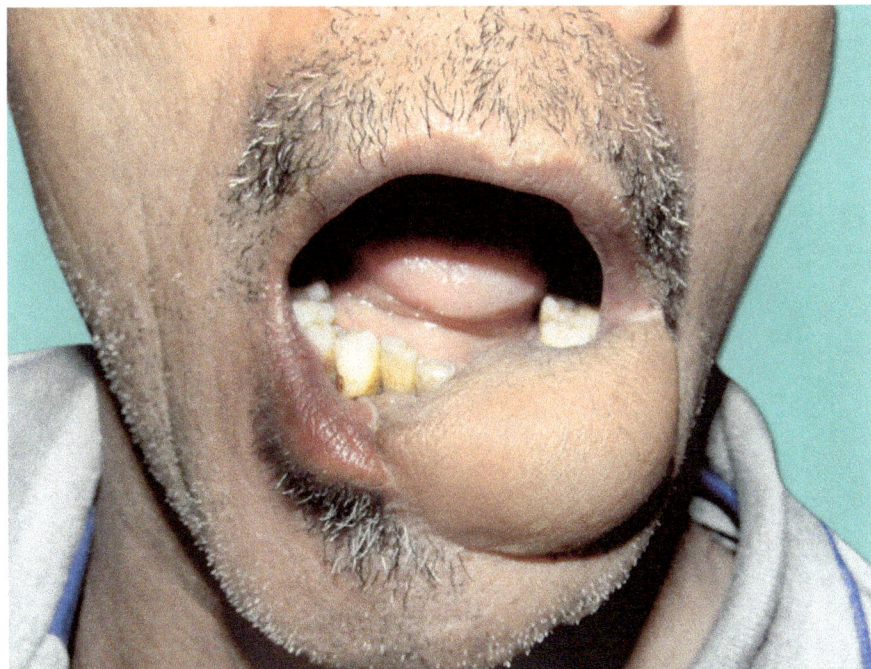

Fig. 18: Follow-up after 18 months.

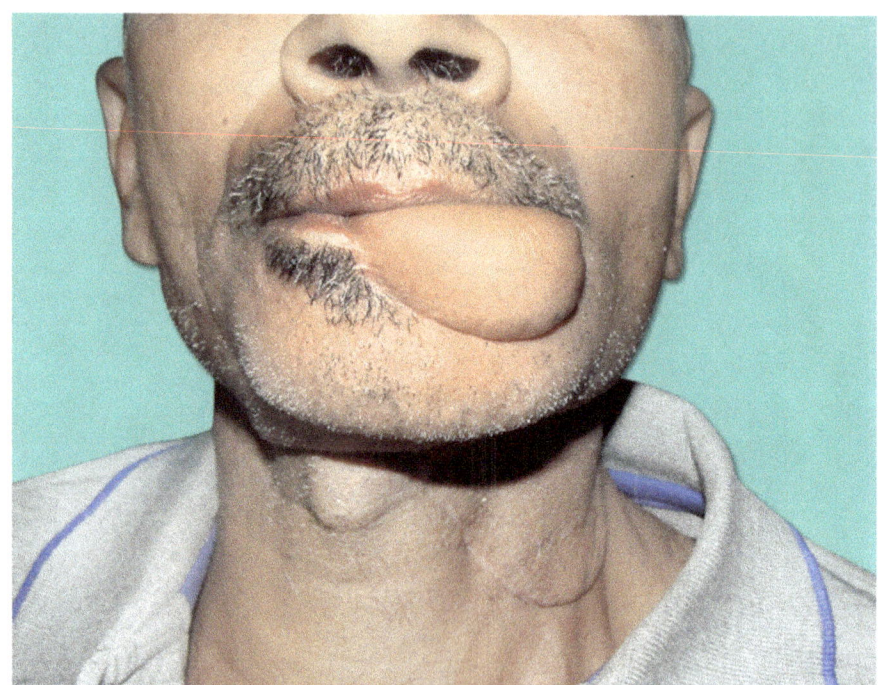

Fig. 19: Very good cosmetic out come after 18 months.

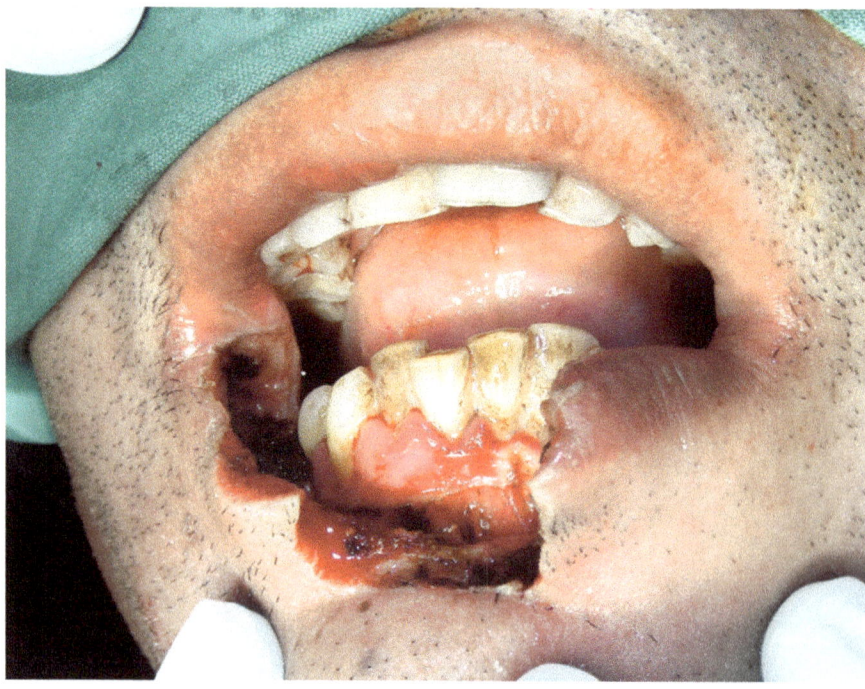

Fig. 20: Carcinoma of lower lip and buccal mucosa excision is done.[1]

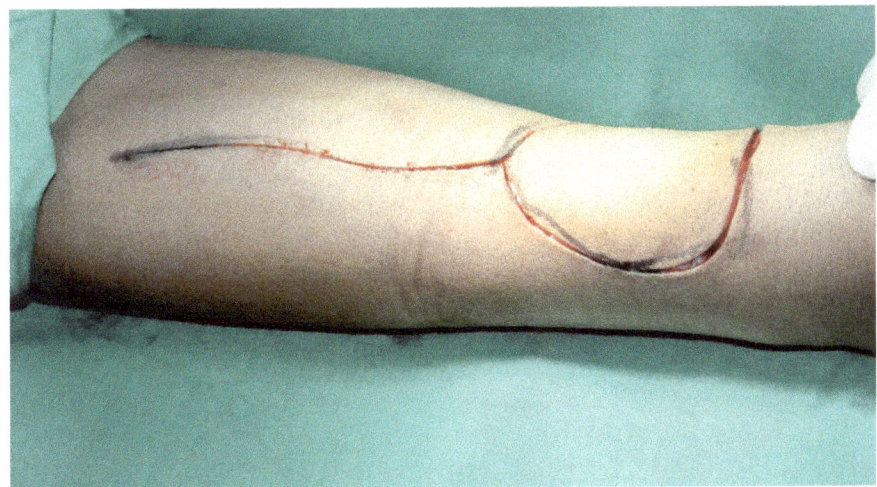

Fig. 21: Incision is kept.

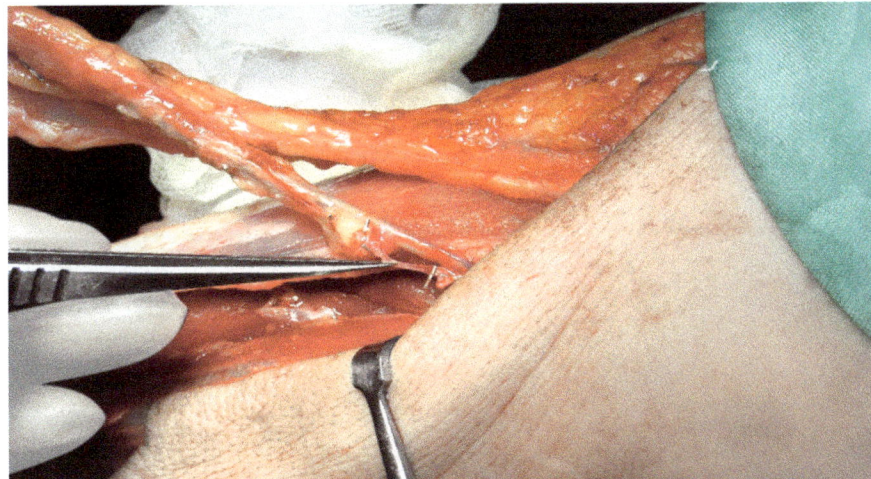

Fig. 22: Flap is raised.

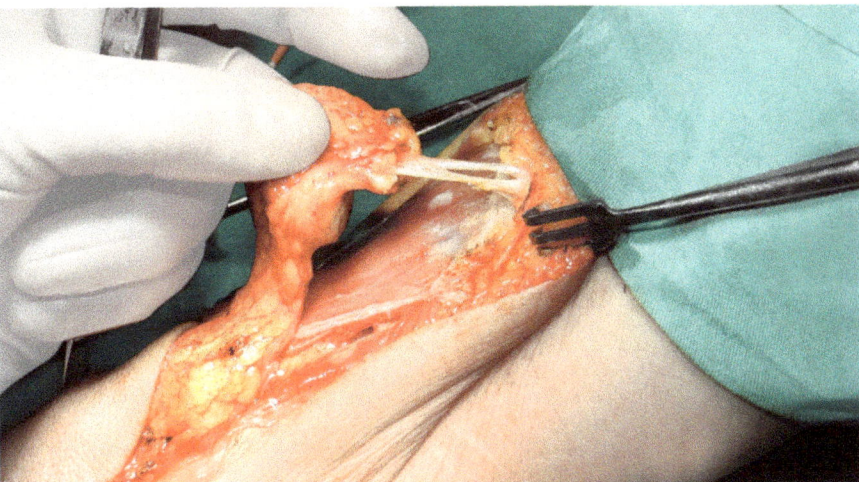

Fig. 23: Vessels seen at elbow.

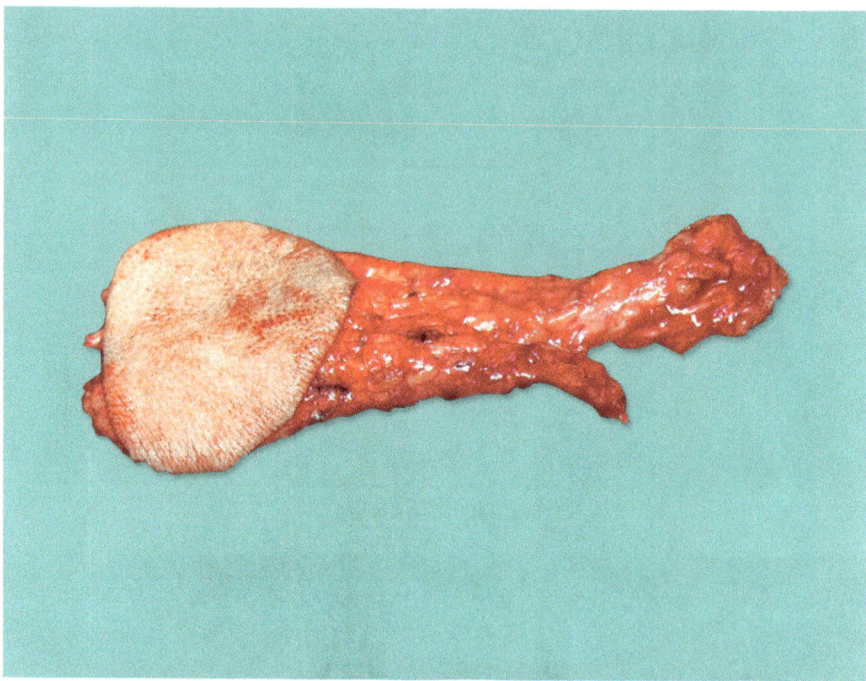

Fig. 24: Flap is divided.

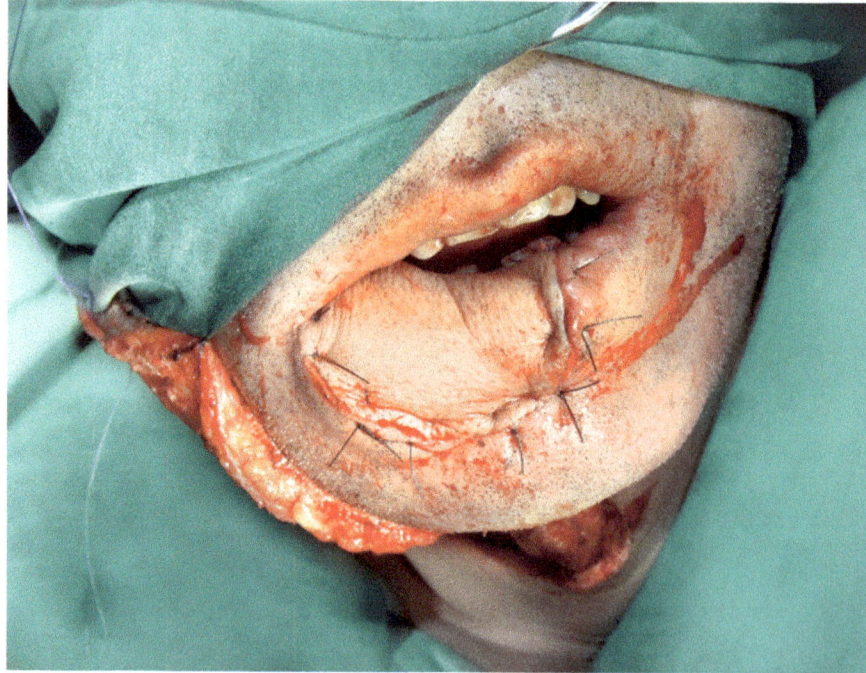

Fig. 25: Inset is completed.

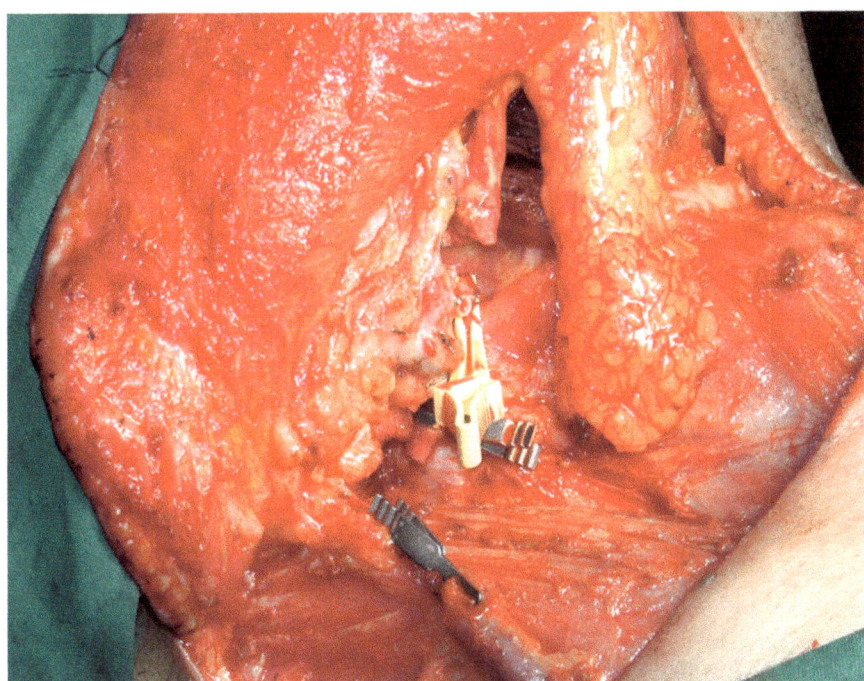

Fig. 26: Vessels are prepared.

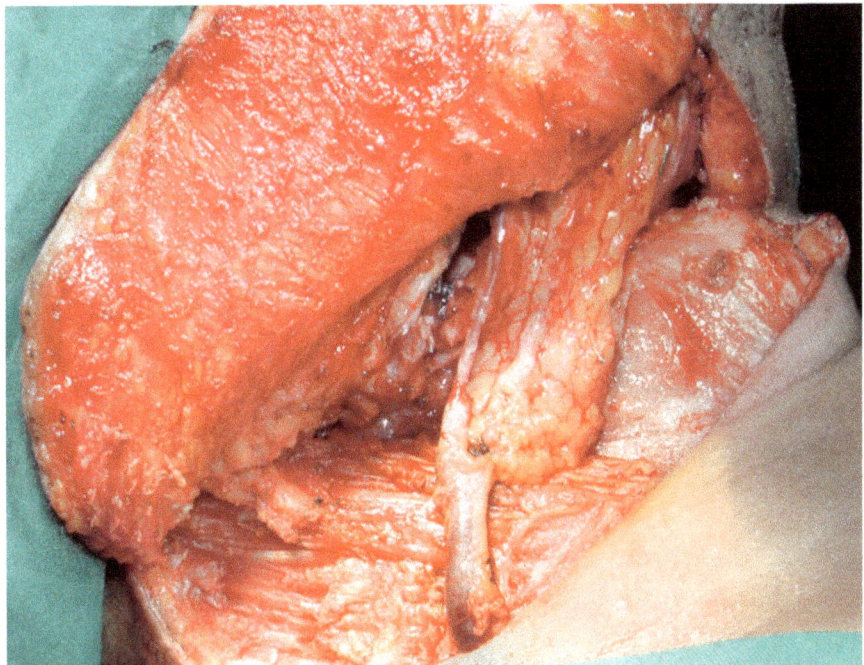

Fig. 27: Facial artery to radial artery, venae comitant to facial vein and cephalic vein to external jugular vein anastomosis were done.

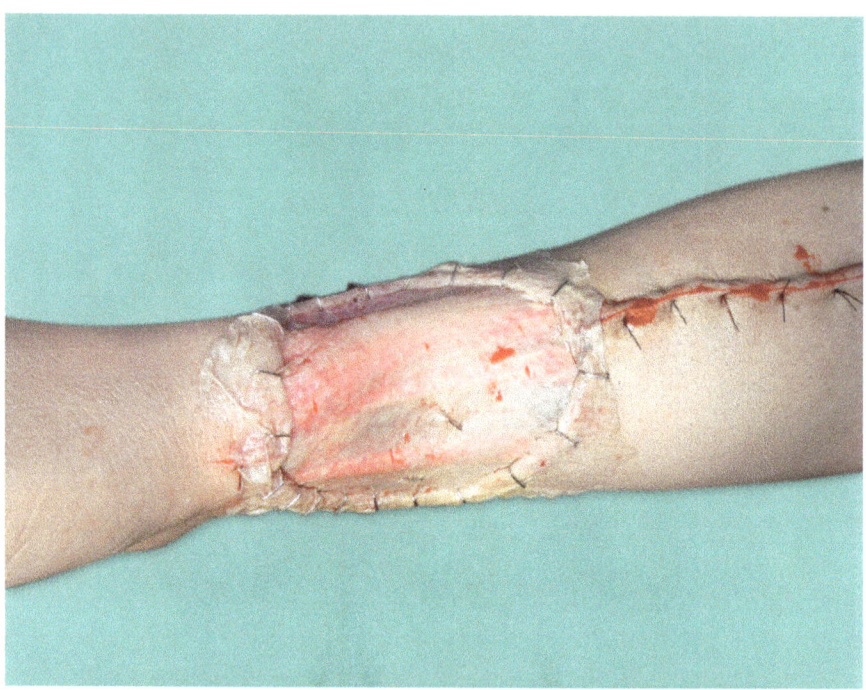

Fig. 28: Donor site is covered with split thickness skin graft.

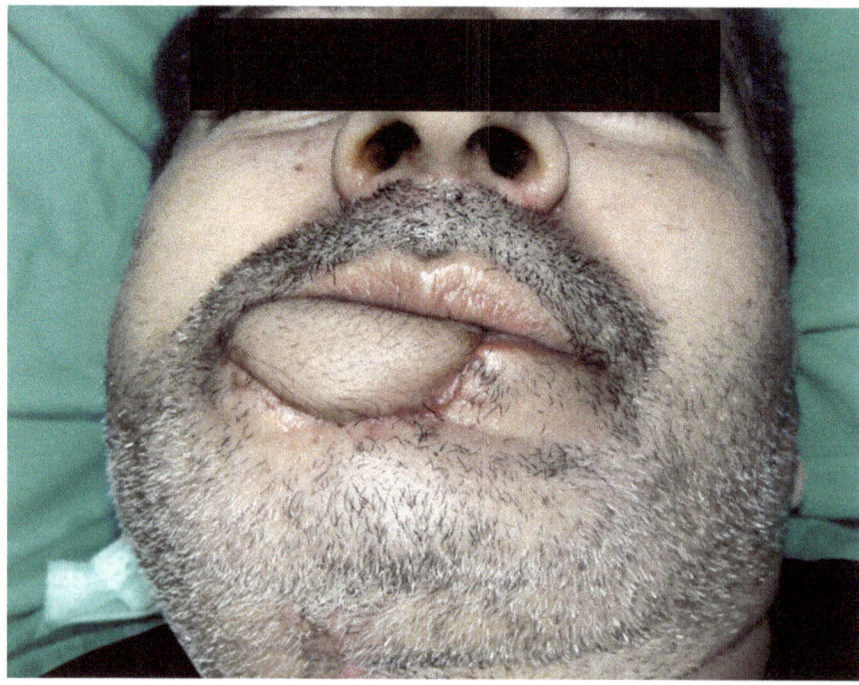

Fig. 29A

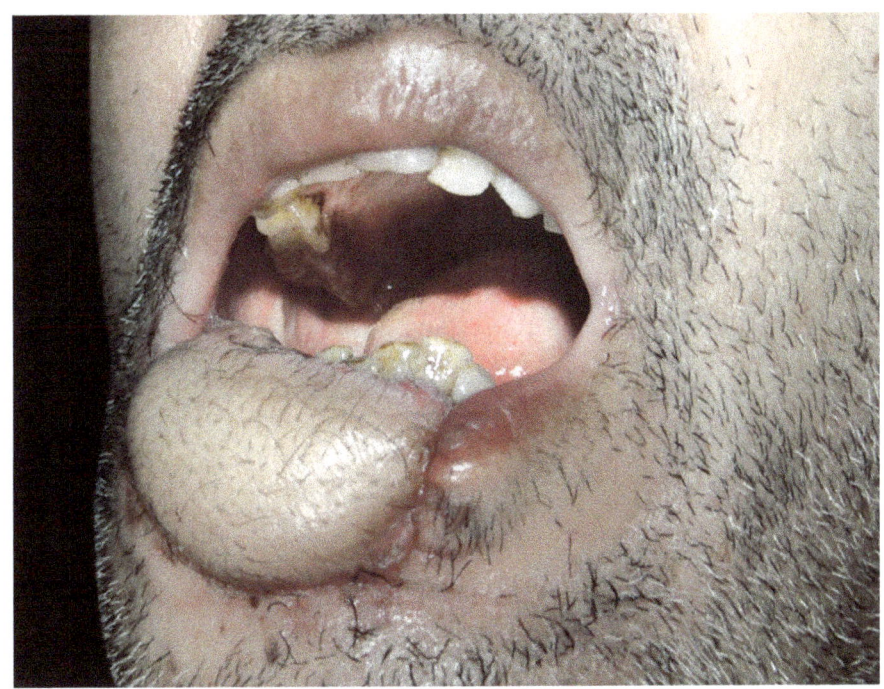

Fig. 29B
Figs. 29A and B: Follow-up after one year.

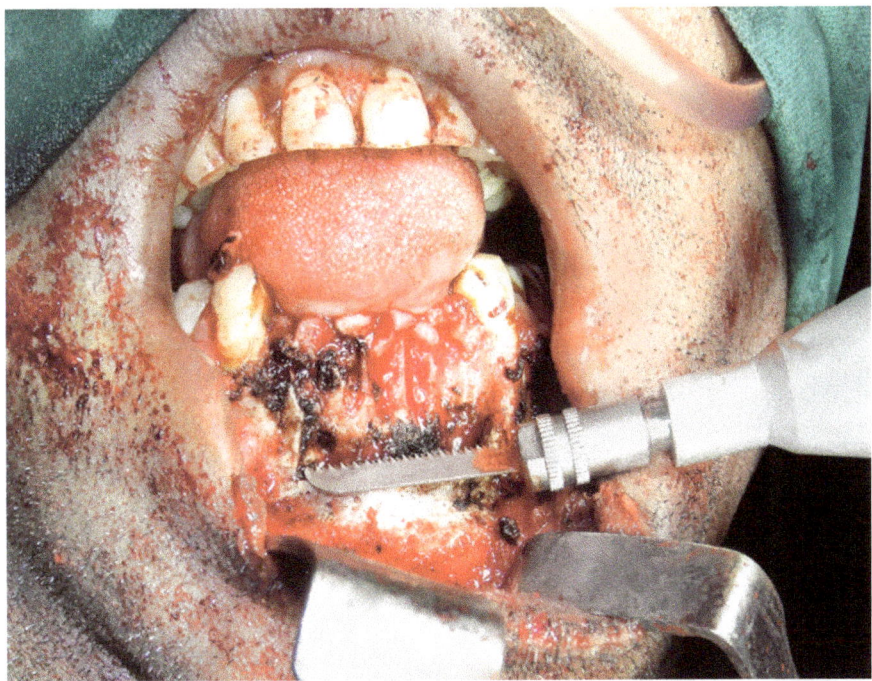

Fig. 30: Carcinoma of lower lip excision and marginal mandibulectomy done.

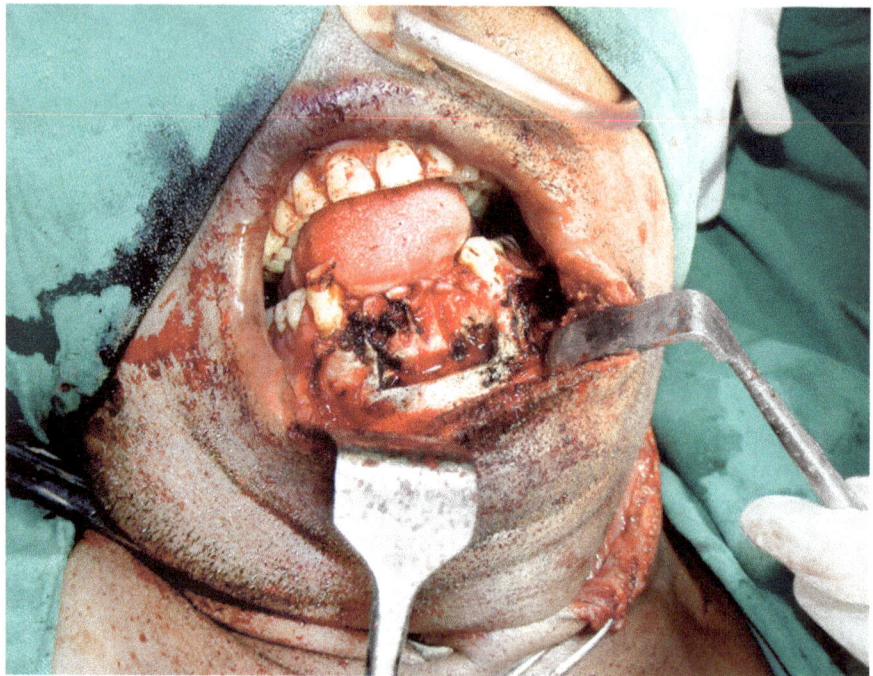

Fig. 31: Marginal mandibulectomy is done.

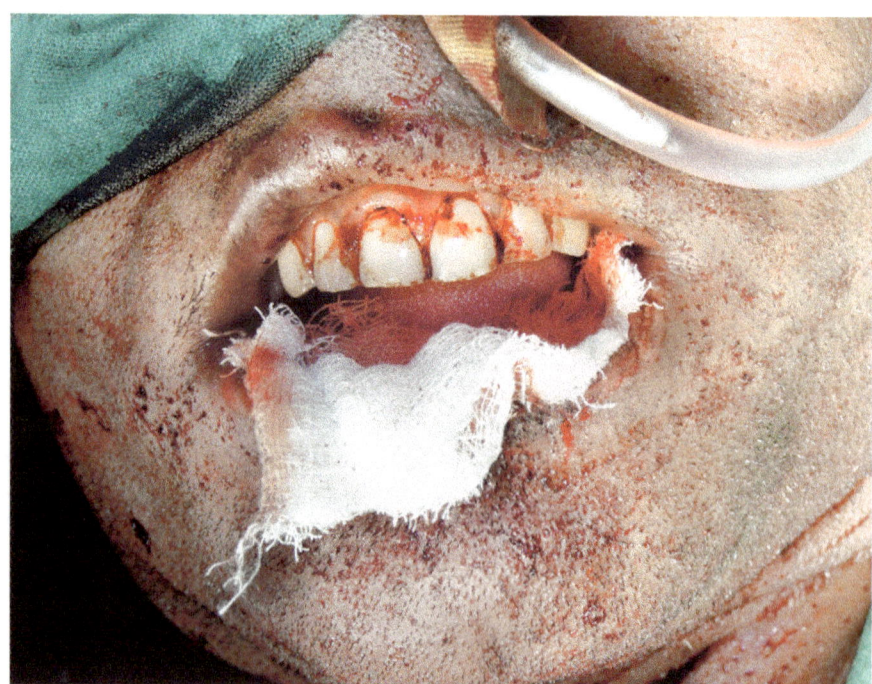

Fig. 32: Measurement is done.

Case Studies

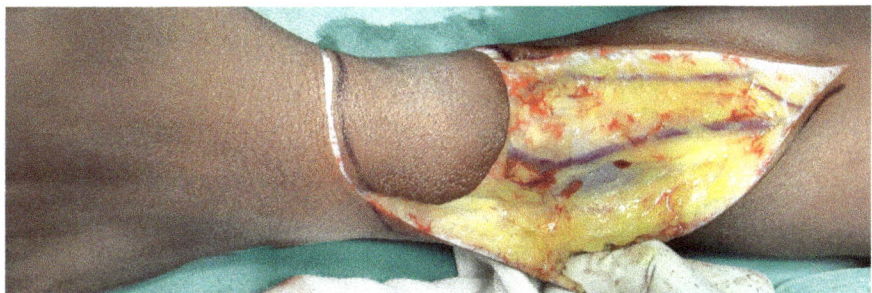

Fig. 33: Flap is raised, cephalic vein is seen.

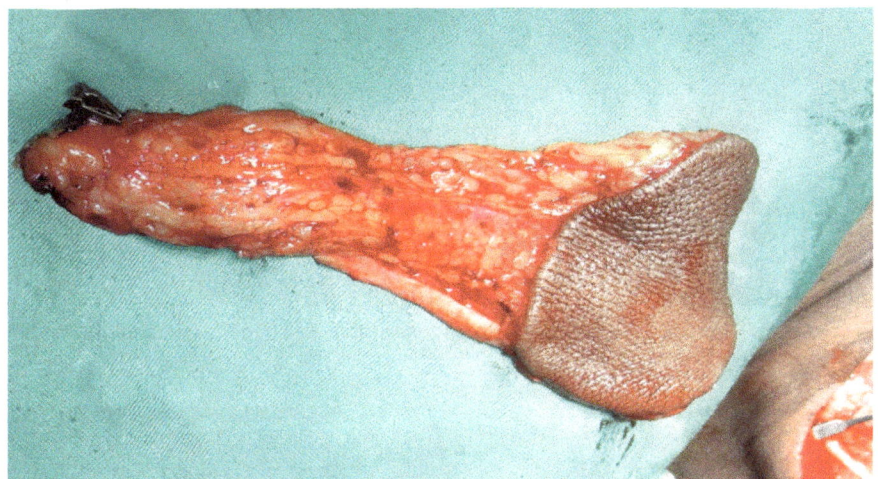

Fig. 34: Flap was harvested with palmaris longus tendon.

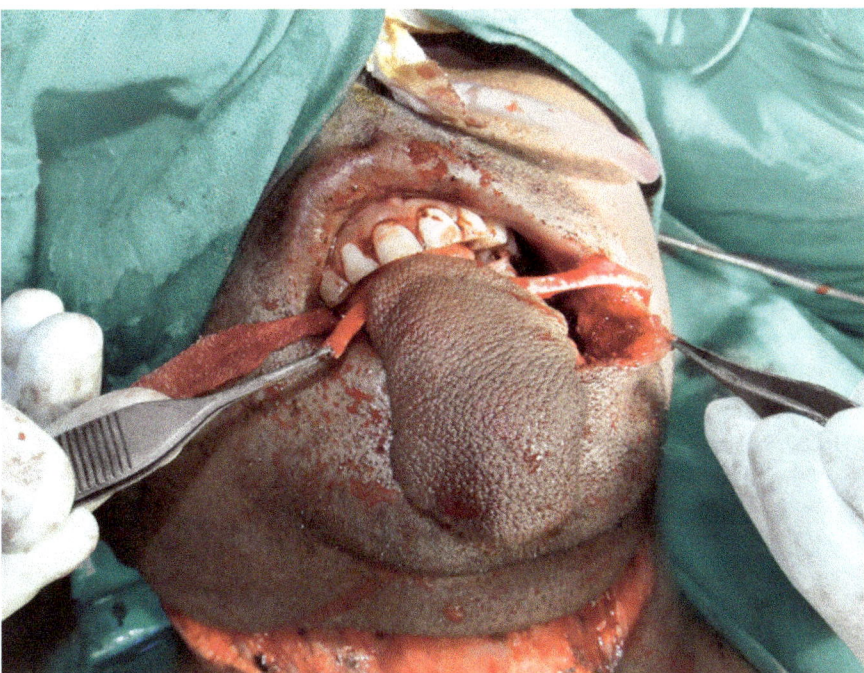

Fig. 35: Palmaris longus is used as a sling for support of lower lip.

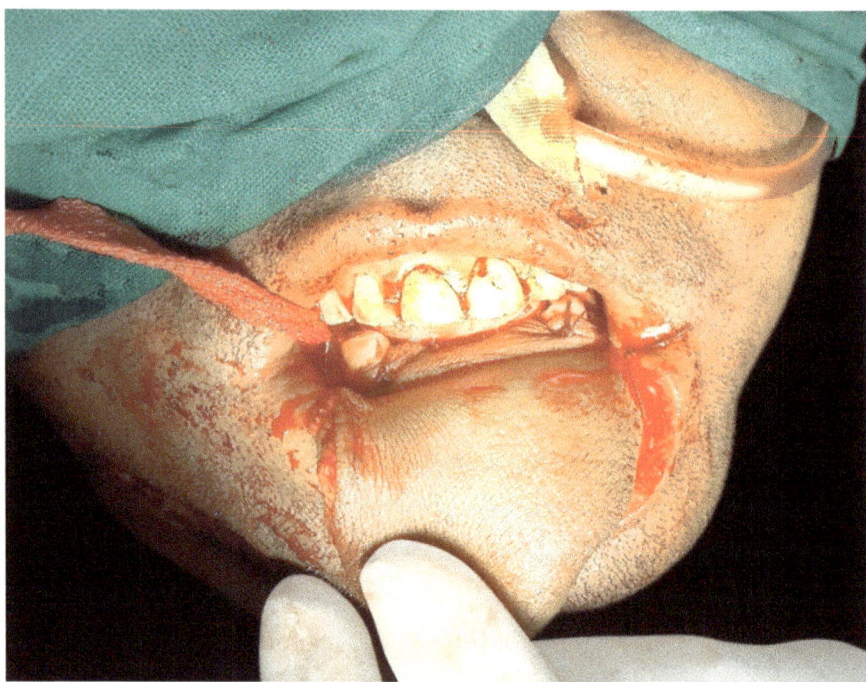

Fig. 36: Palmaris longus is sutured with orbicularis oris muscle and flap is sutured to mucosal lining.

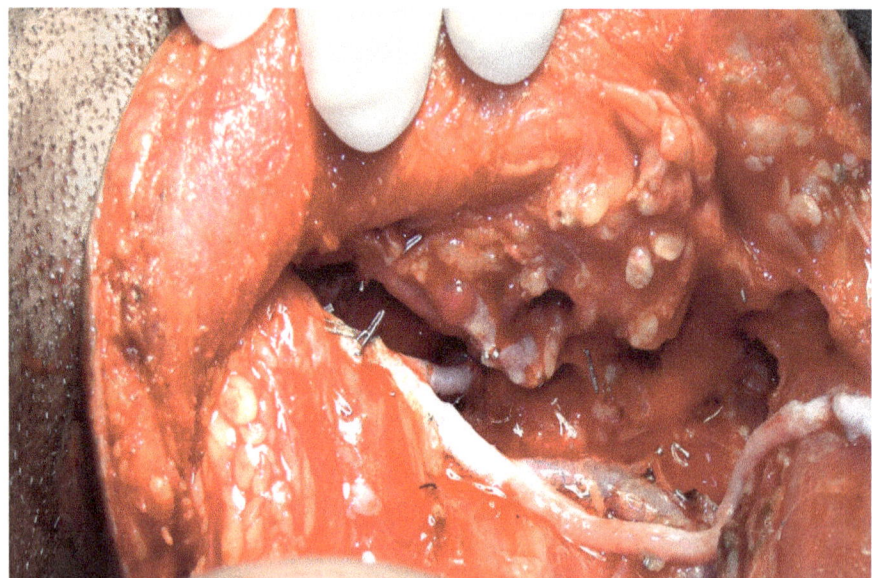

Fig. 37: Radial artery was anastomosed to facial artery, cephalic vein was anastomosed to common facial vein and venae comitant was anastomosed to external jugular vein with interpositional saphenous vein graft.

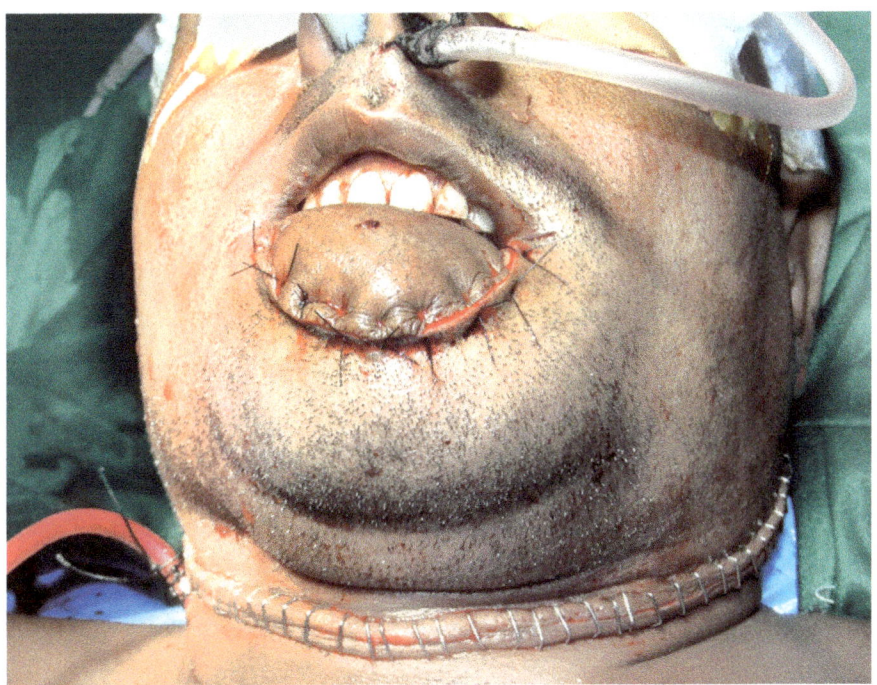

Fig. 38: Hemostasis is done, drain is kept away from anastomosis site and neck is sutured layerwise.

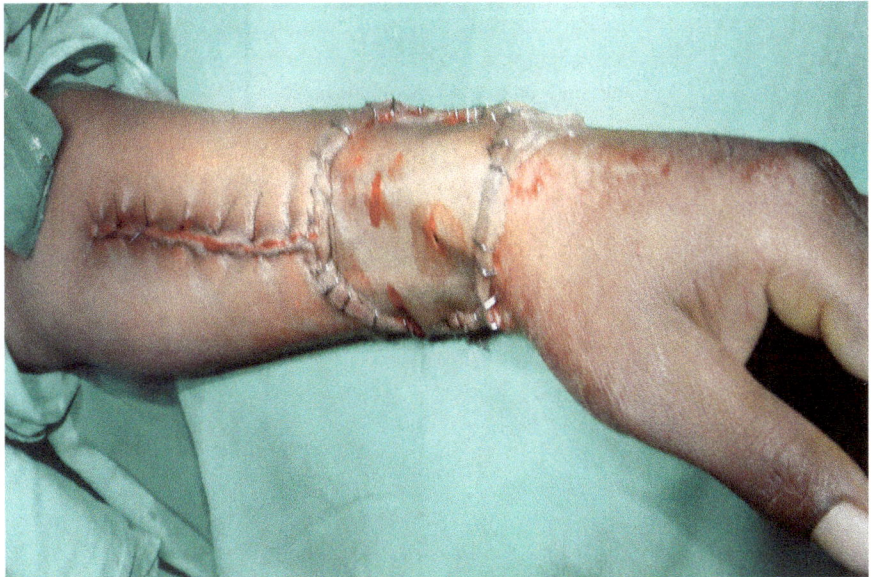

Fig. 39: Donor site is covered with split thickness skin graft.

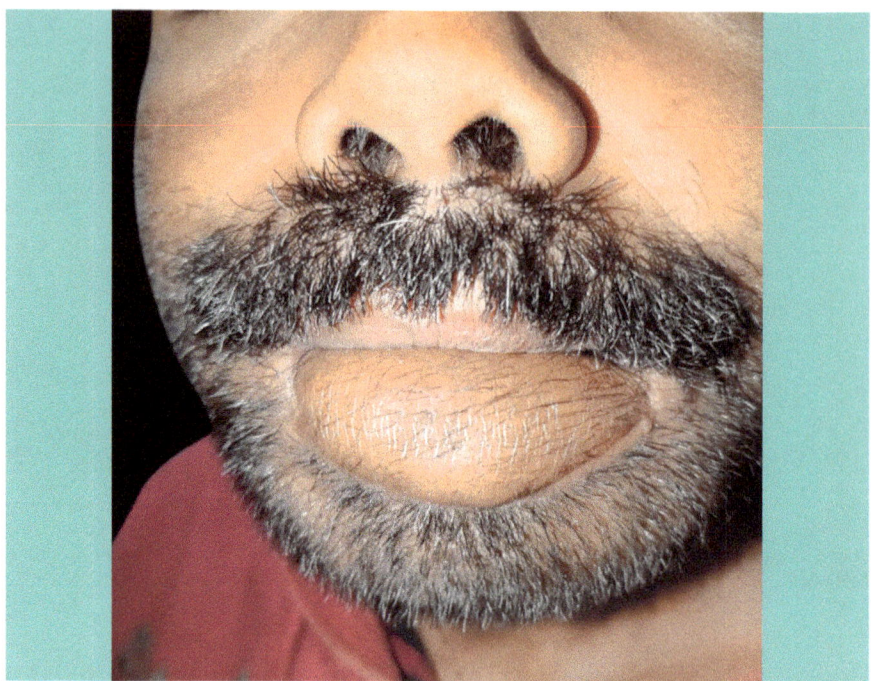

Fig. 40: Follow-up after 18 months.[2]

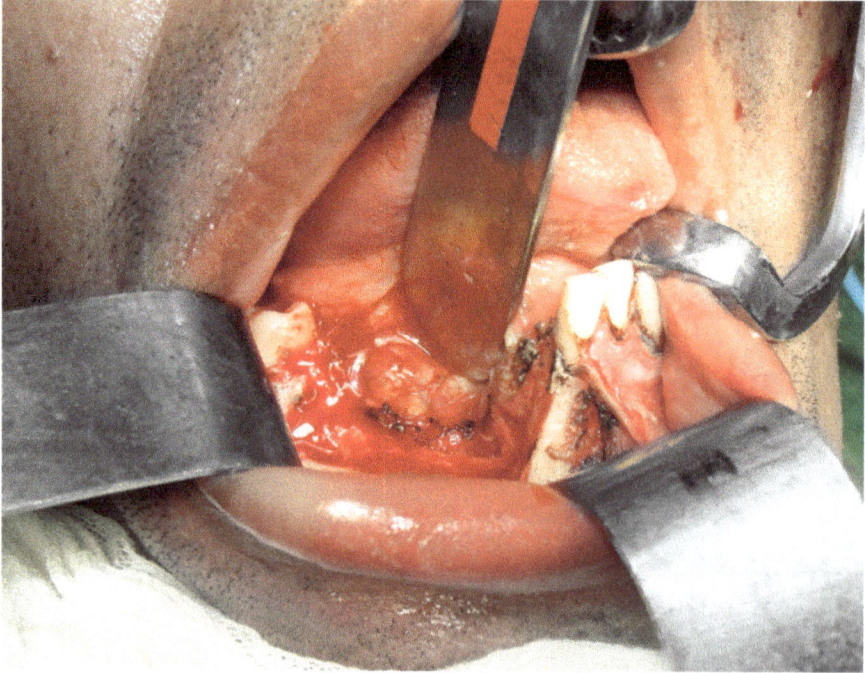

Fig. 41: Carcinoma of lower lip mucosa excision and marginal mandibulectomy is done.

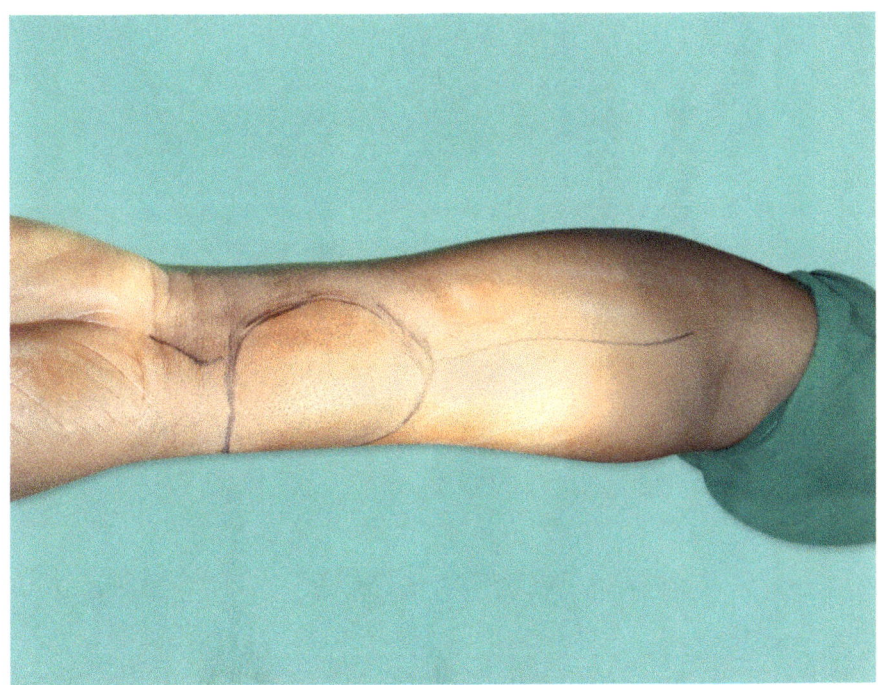

Fig. 42: Marking is done.

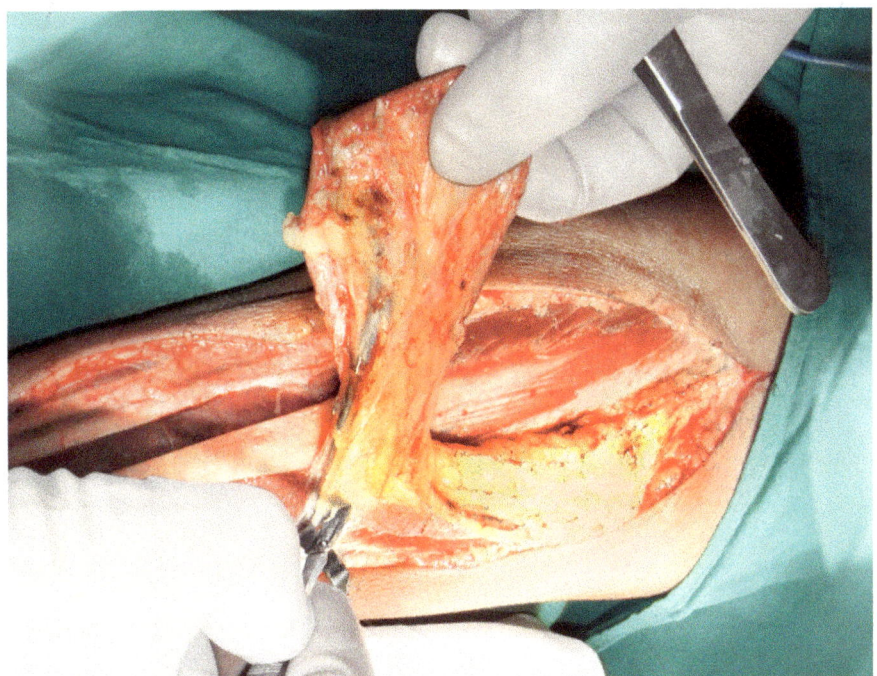

Fig. 43: Flap is raised.

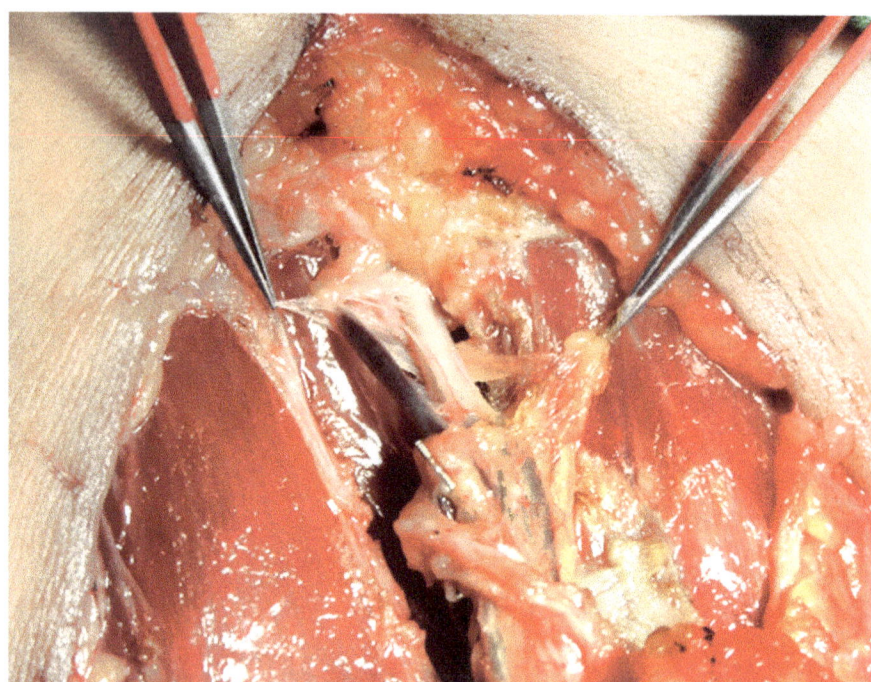

Fig. 44: Radial artery and venae comitantes are separated at elbow.

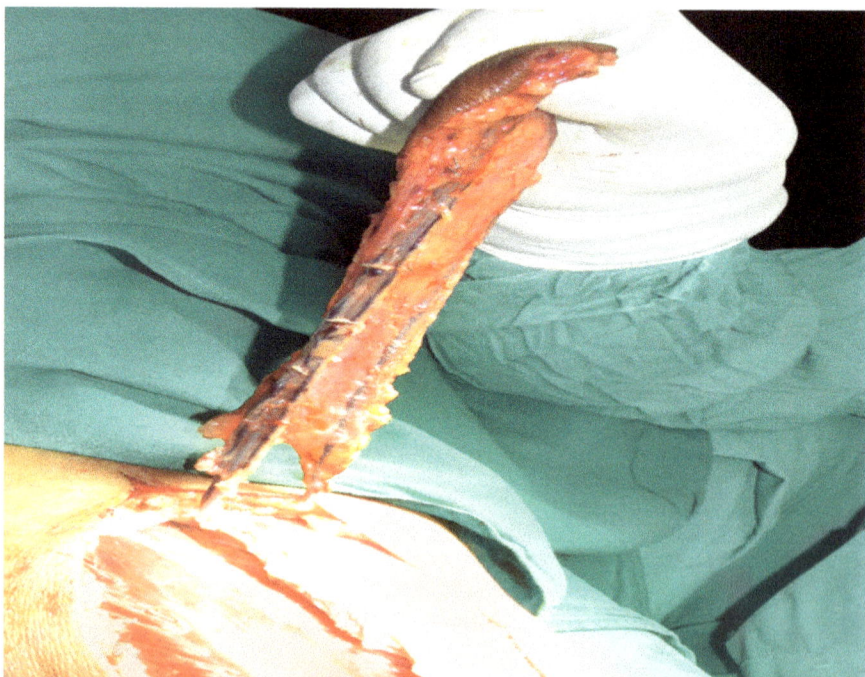

Fig. 45: Flap is raised.

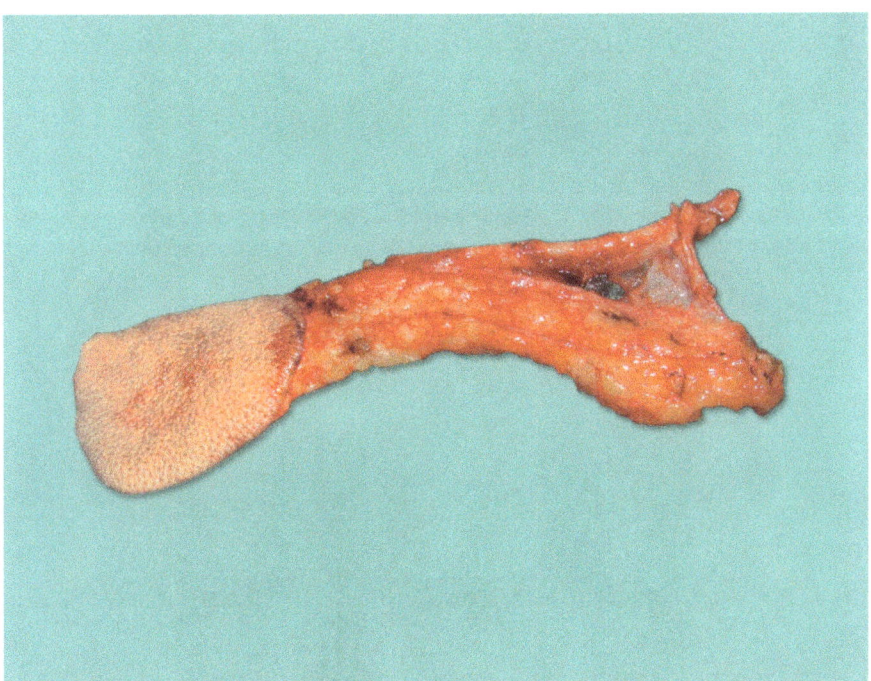

Fig. 46: Flap is harvested.

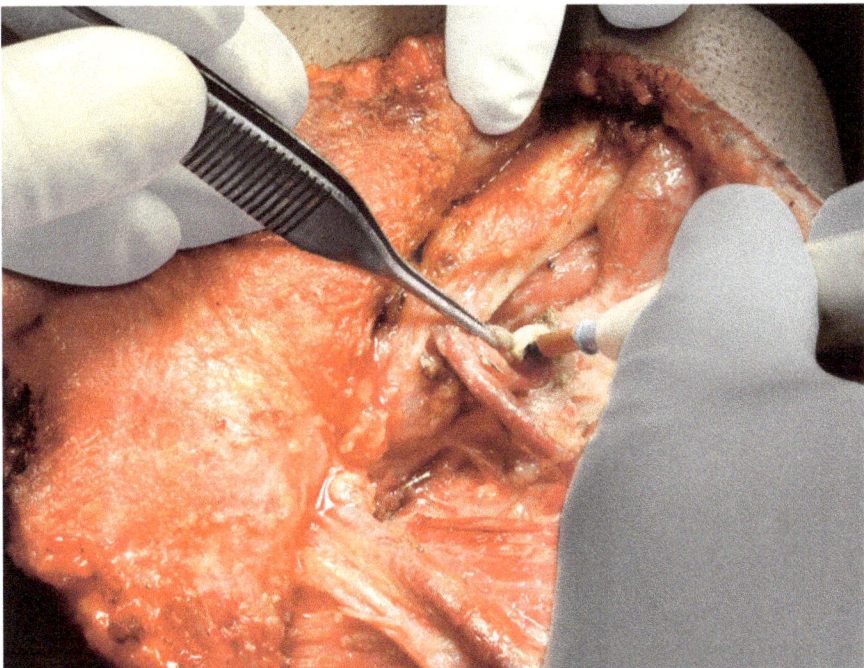

Fig. 47: Digastric muscle and tendon are cut to expose proximal part of facial artery with better blood flow.

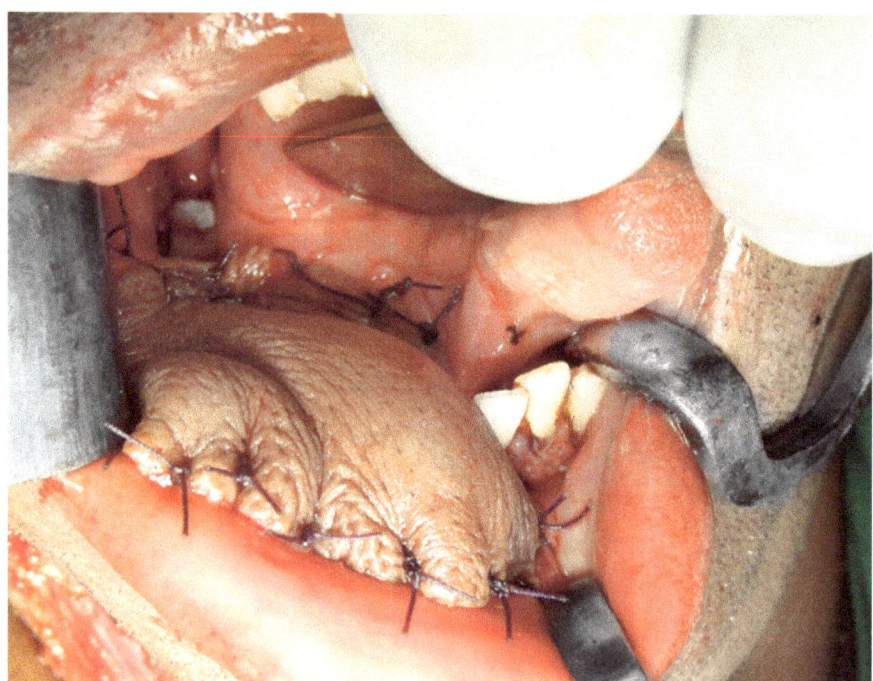

Fig. 48: Inset is given with 2-0 vicryl.

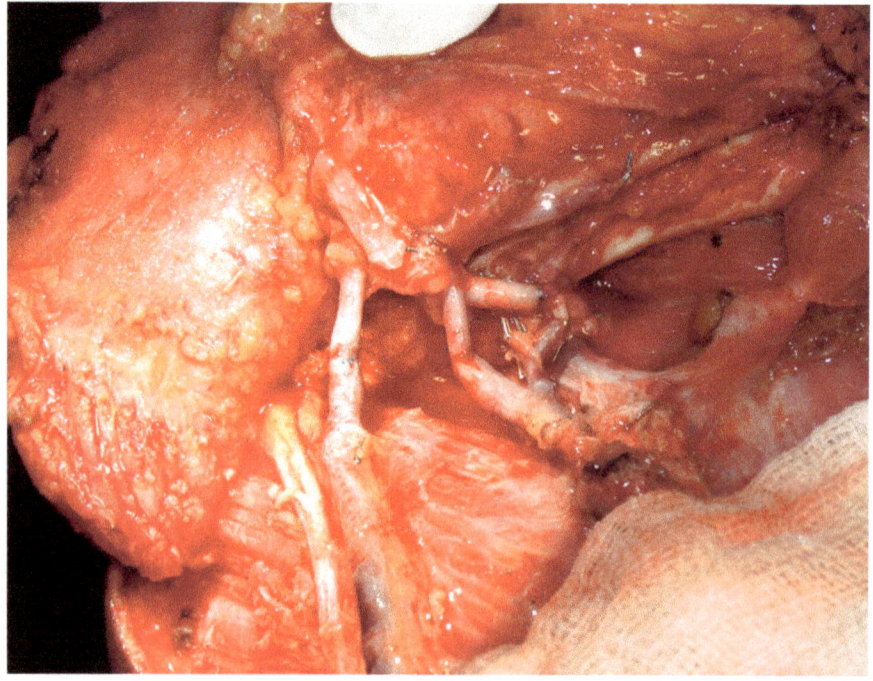

Fig. 49: Radial artery anastomosed to facial artery, venae comitant to facial vein and cephalic vein to external jugular vein.

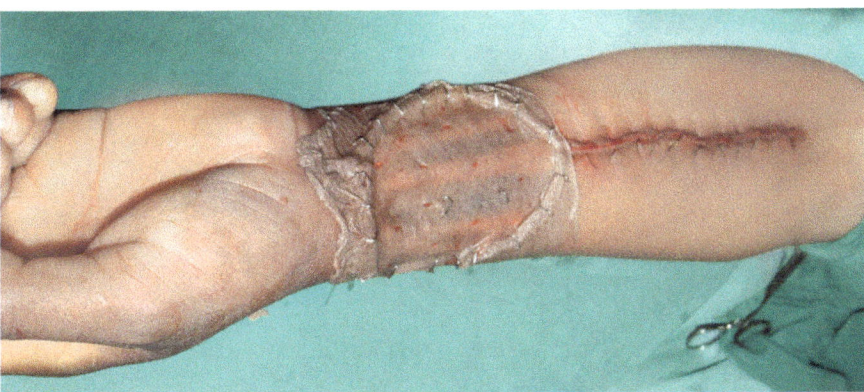
Fig. 50: Donor site.

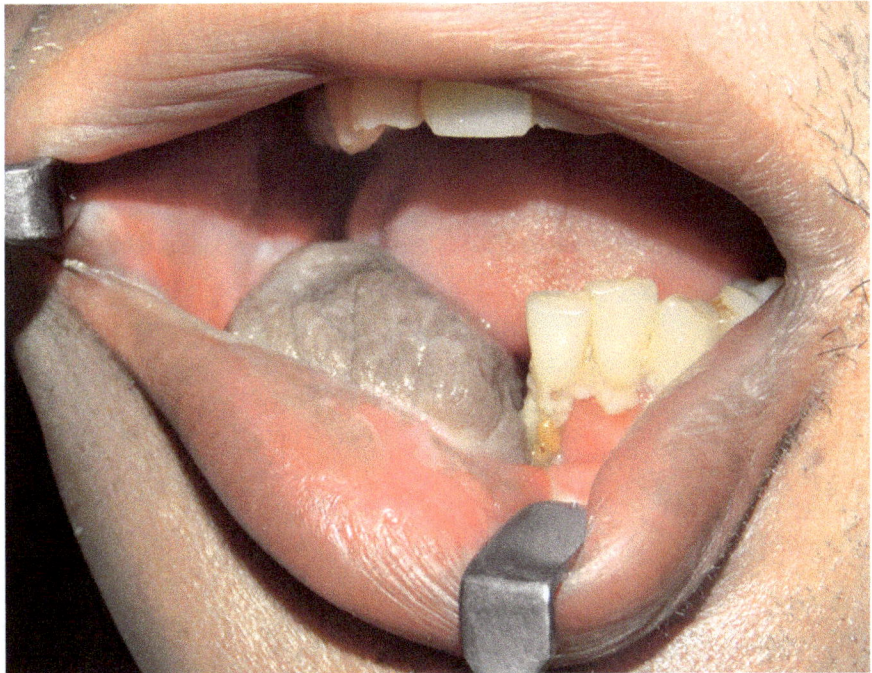
Fig. 51: Follow-up after 15 months.

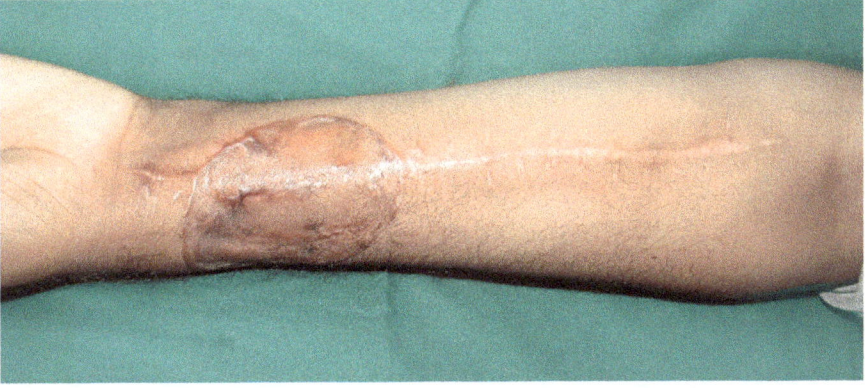
Fig. 52: Good cosmetic outcome of donor site.

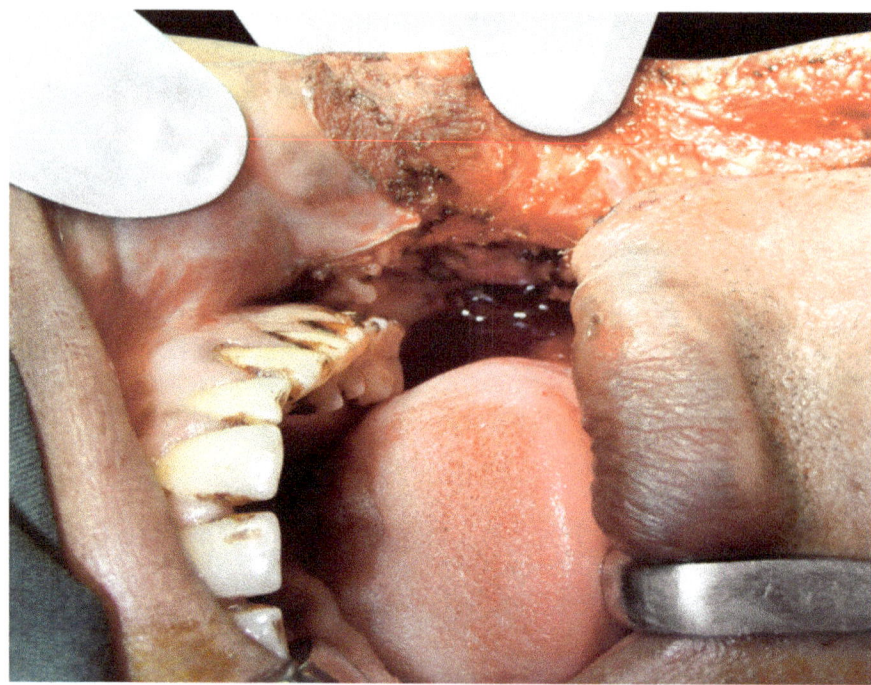

Fig. 53: Carcinoma of left buccal mucosa excision done.

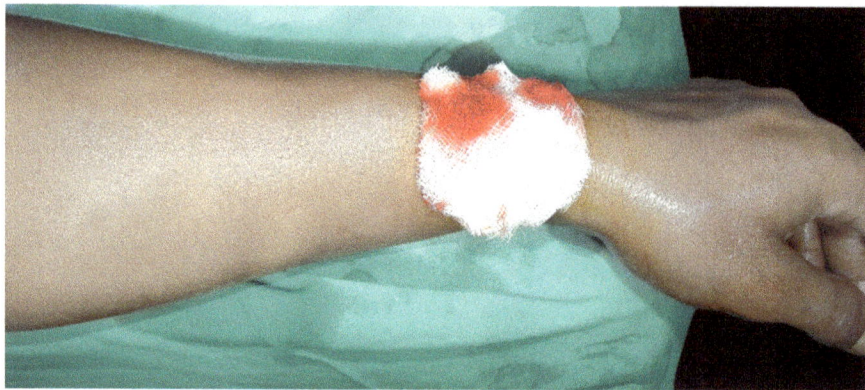

Fig. 54: Measurement is done.

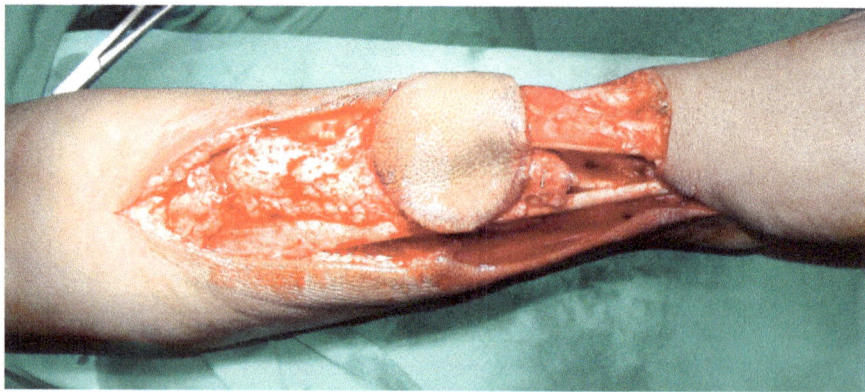

Fig. 55: Flap is raised.

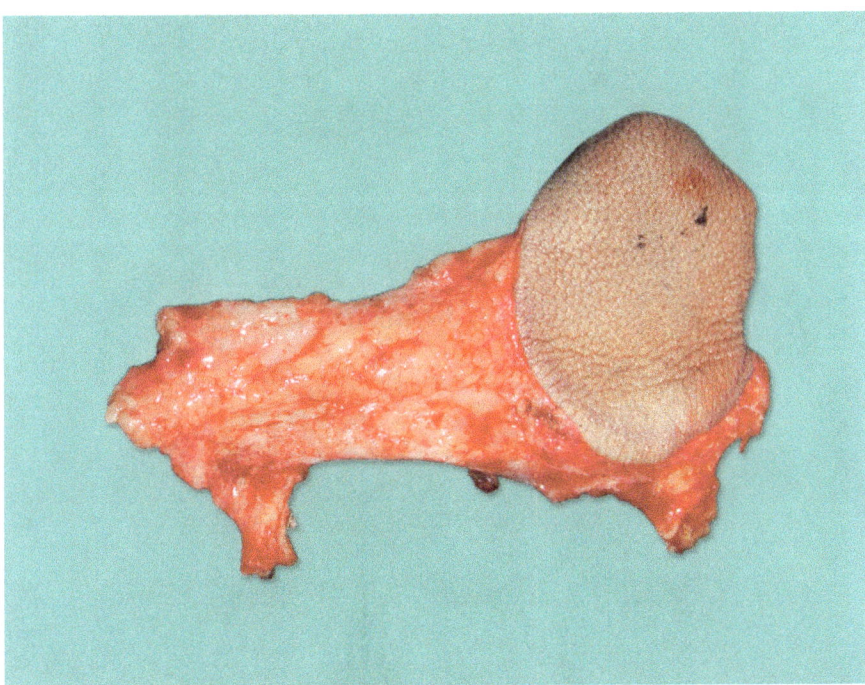

Fig. 56: Flap is harvested.

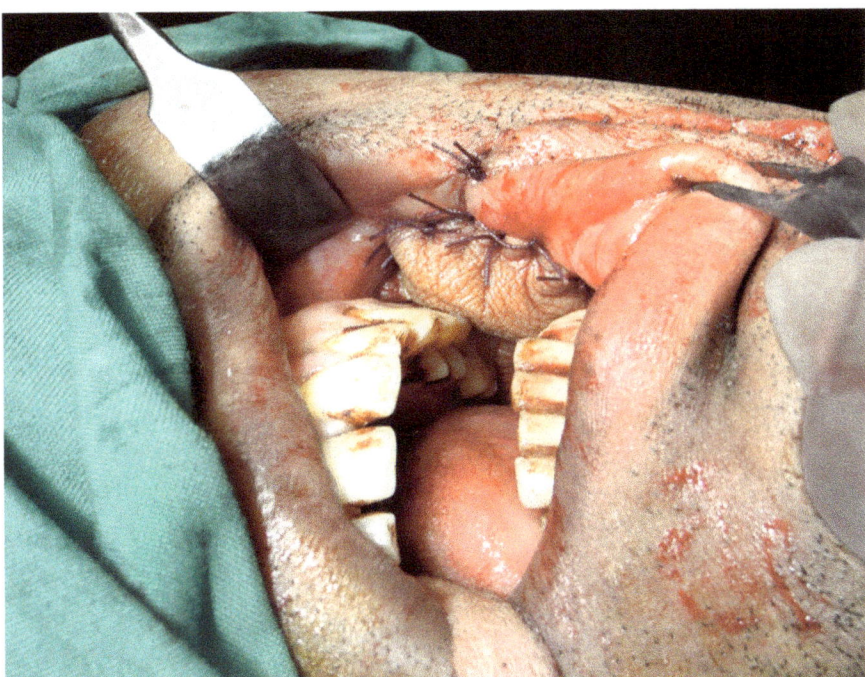

Fig. 57: Inset completed.

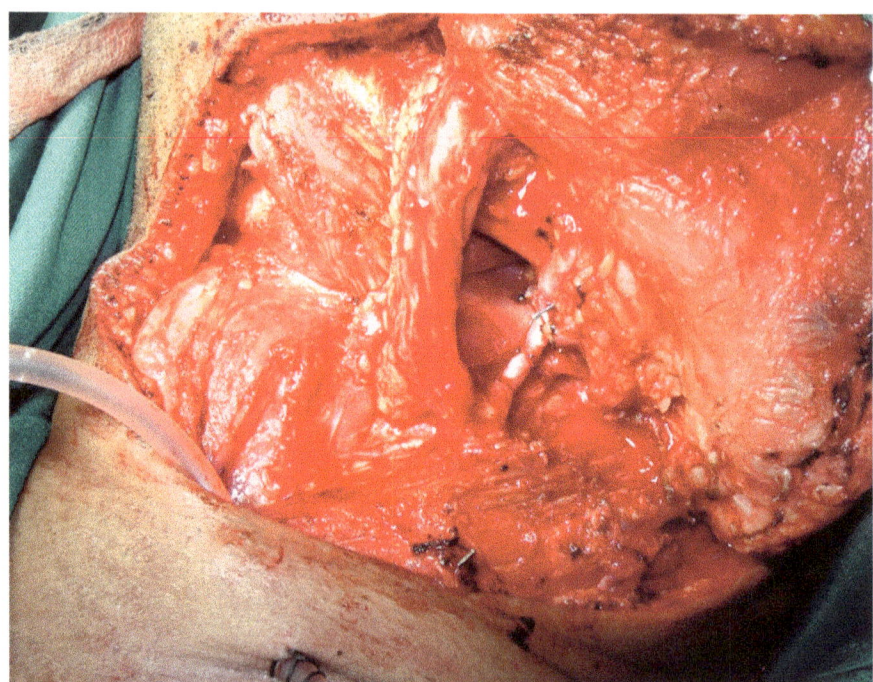

Fig. 58: Radial artery to facial artery, venae comitant to facial vein and cephalic vein to external jugular vein are anastomosed.

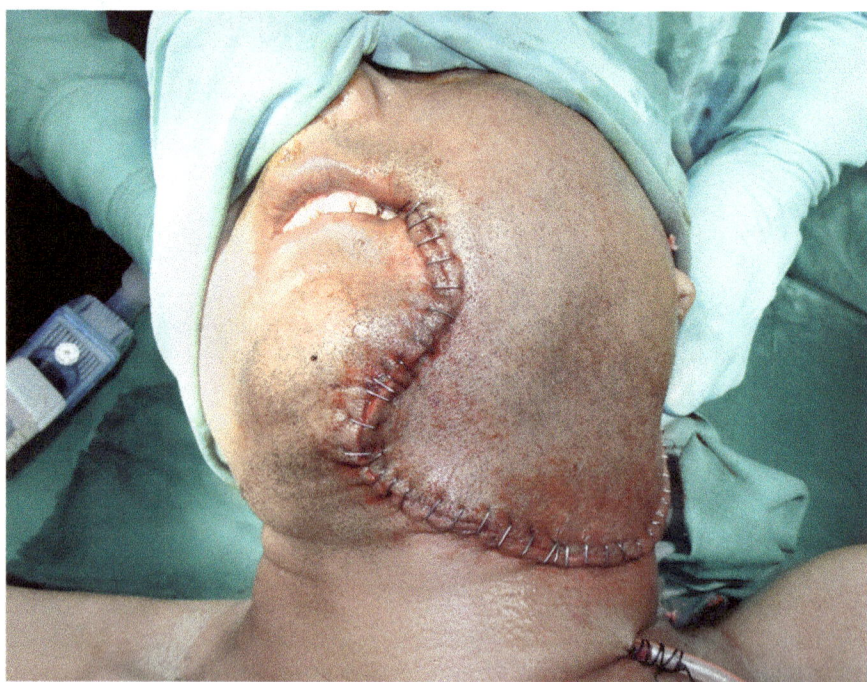

Fig. 59: Final suturing.

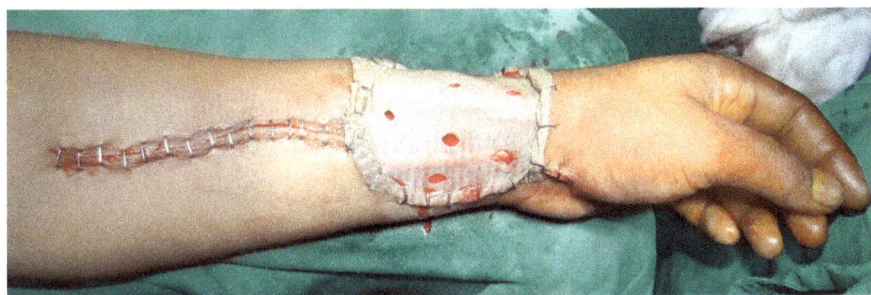

Fig. 60: Donor site.

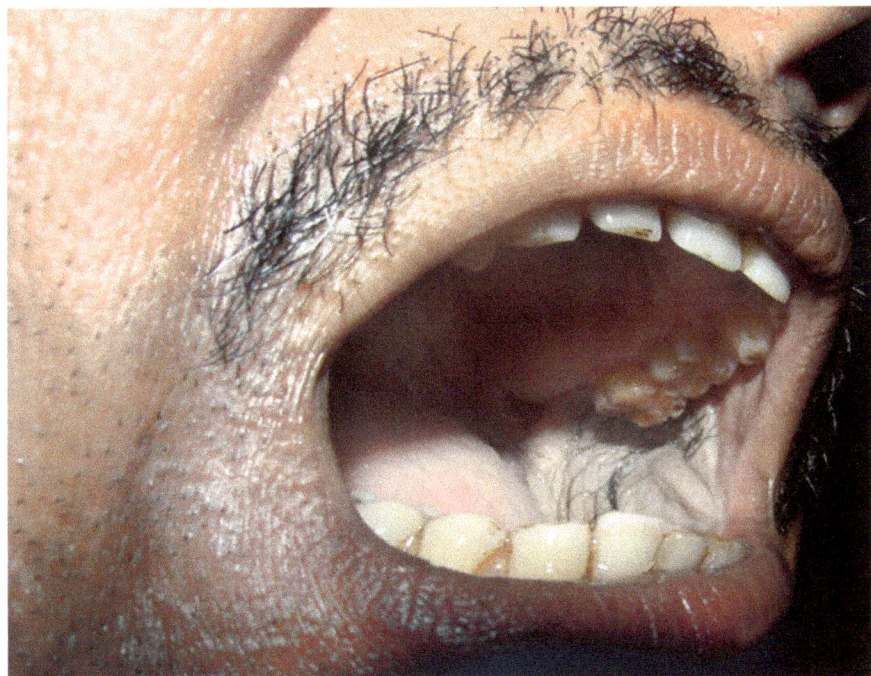

Fig. 61: Follow-up after 14 months with excellent mouth opening.[3]

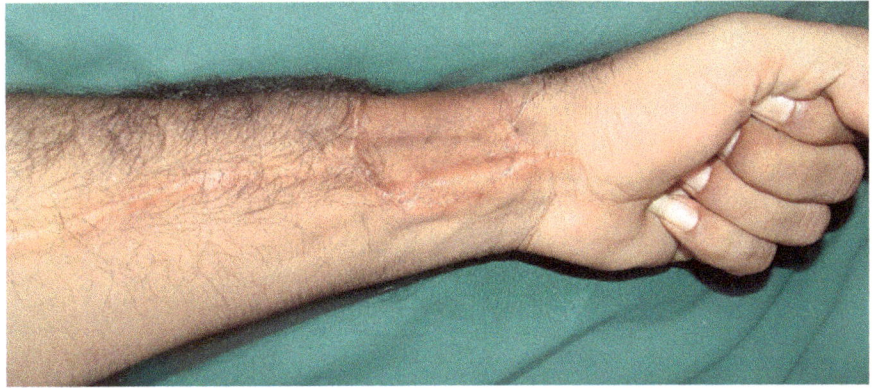

Fig. 62: Excellent cosmetic outcome of donor site.

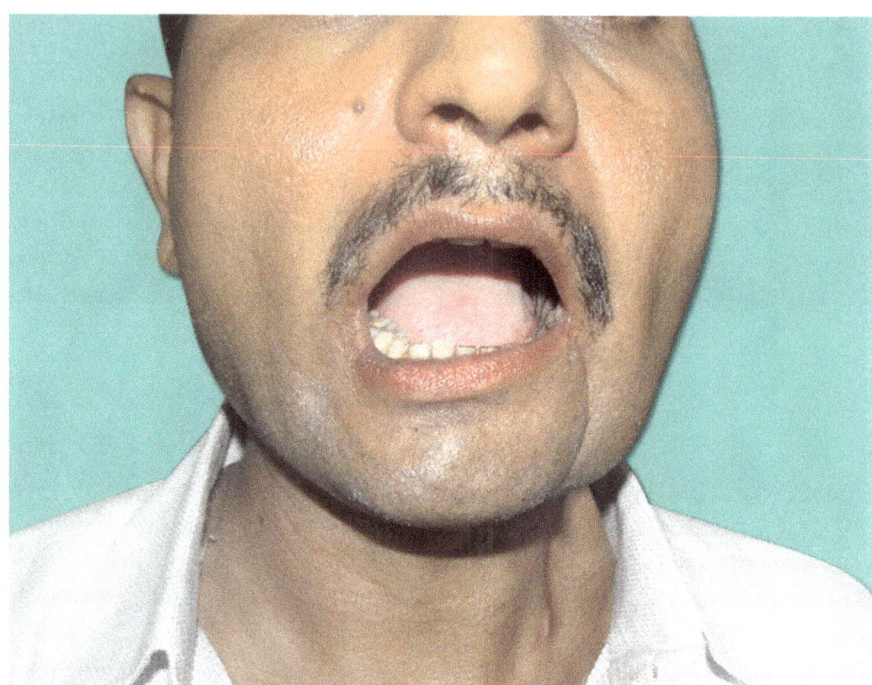

Fig. 63: Three and half fingers mouth opening.

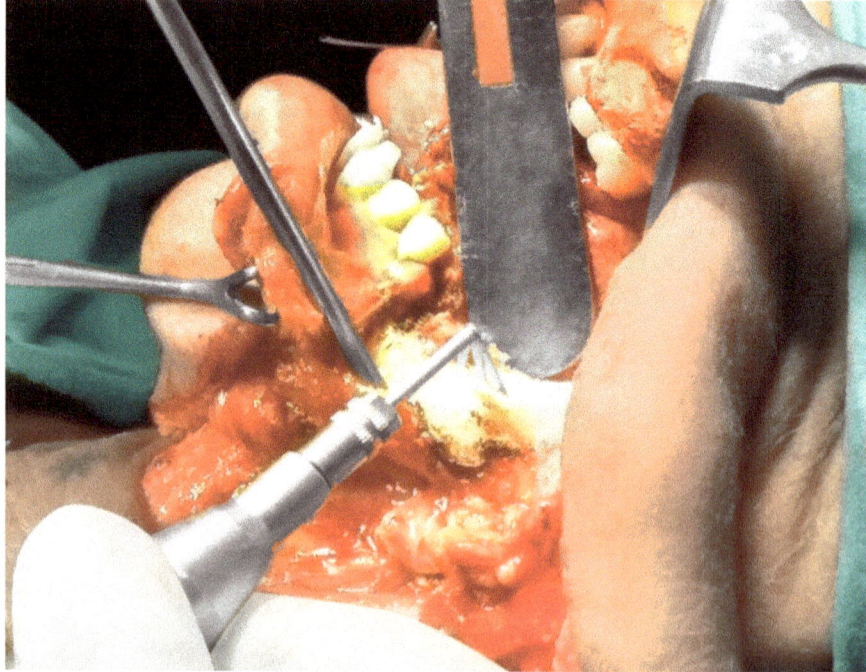

Fig. 64: Marginal mandibulectomy is done.

Case Studies

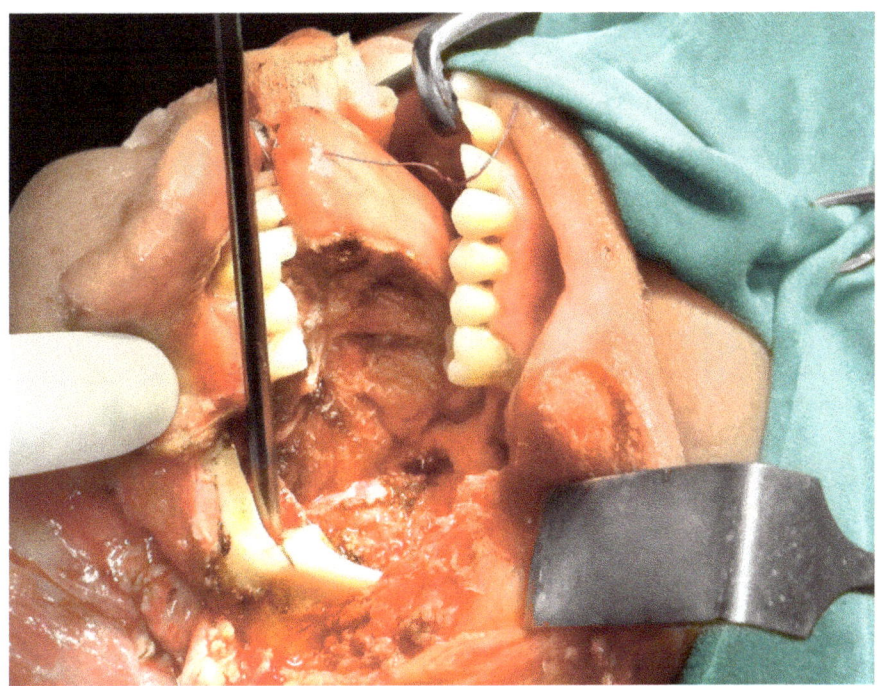

Fig. 65: About 70% of the tongue was excised.[4]

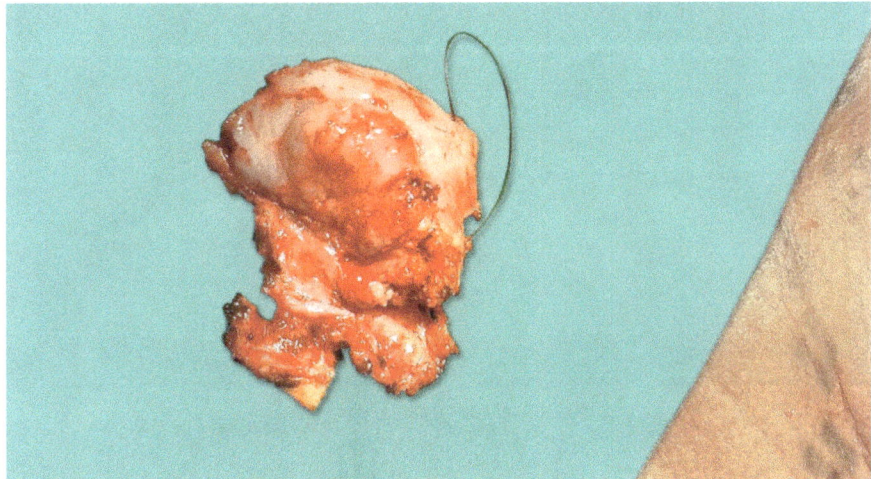

Fig. 66: Excised specimen.

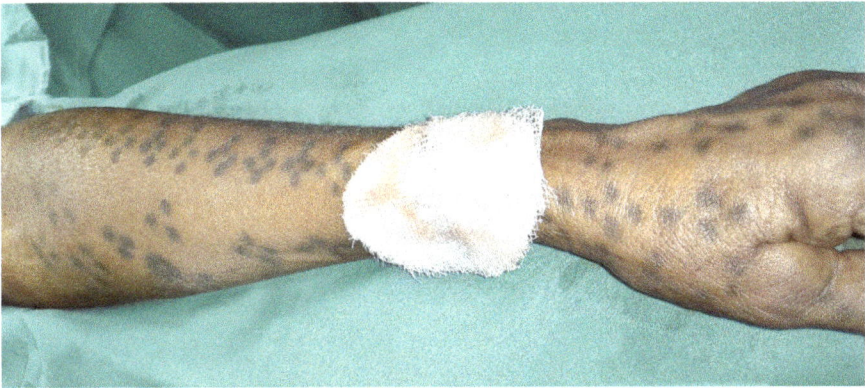

Fig. 67: Measurement is done.

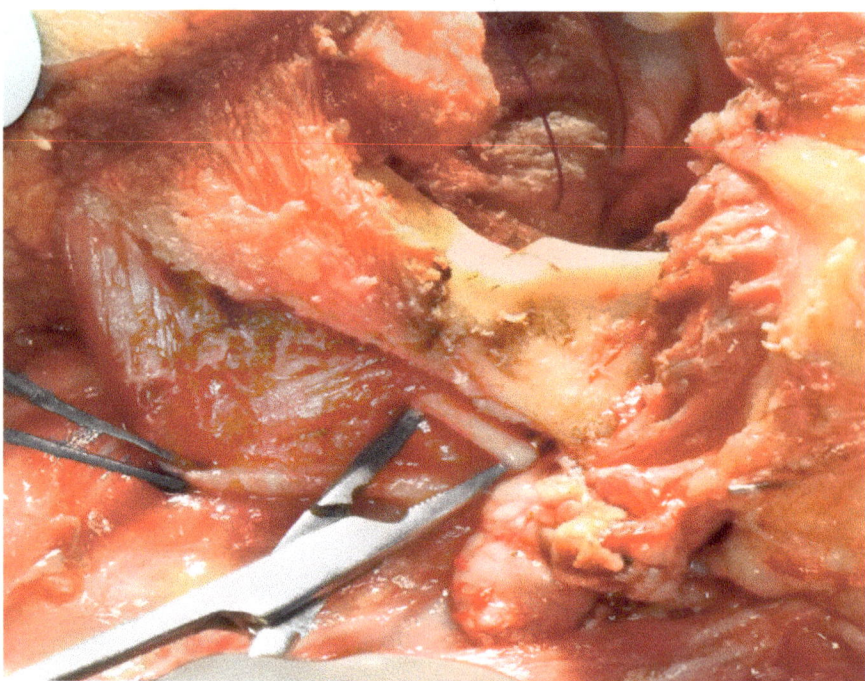

Fig. 68: Lingual nerve is dissected.

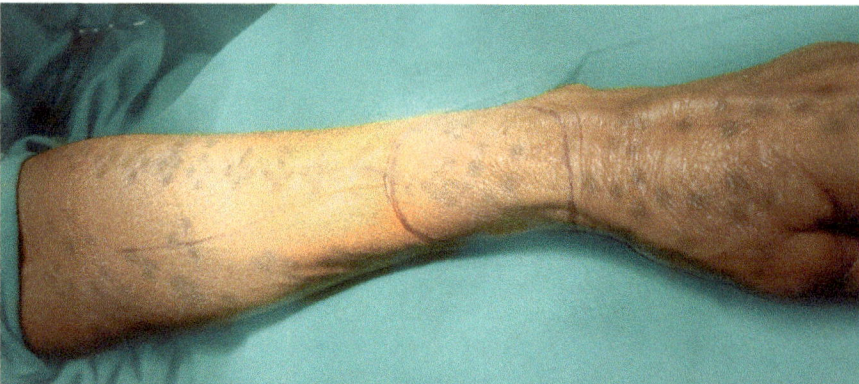

Fig. 69: Marking of flap is done.

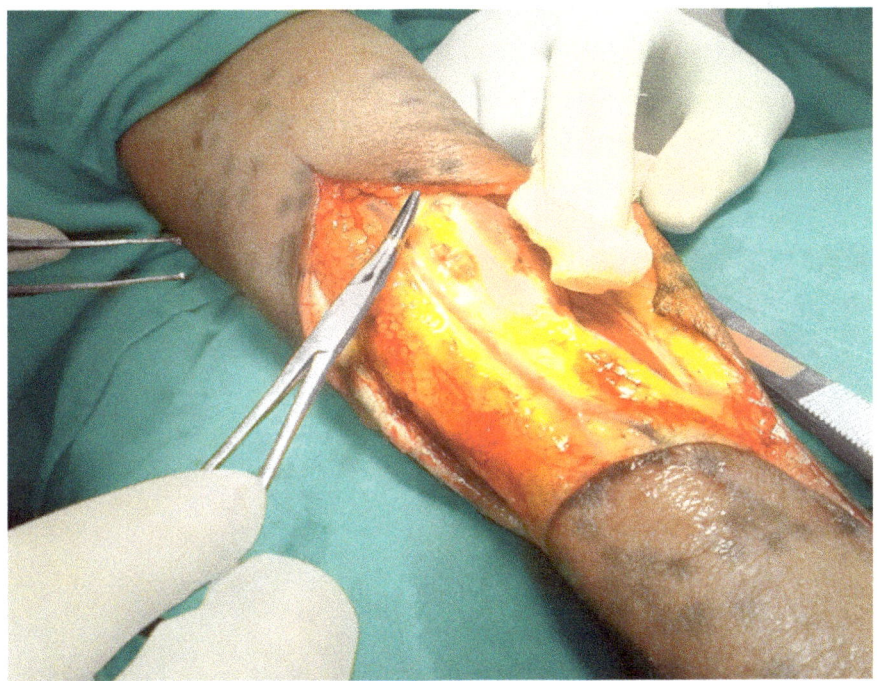
Fig. 70: Lateral antebrachial nerve is dissected.

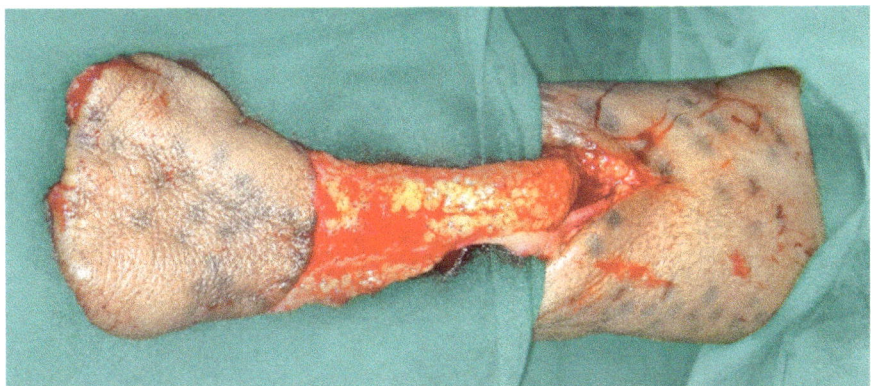
Fig. 71: Flap is raised.

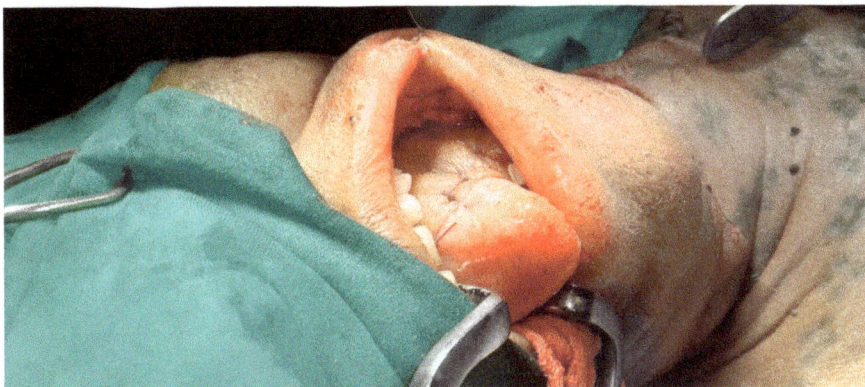
Fig. 72: Inset is given.

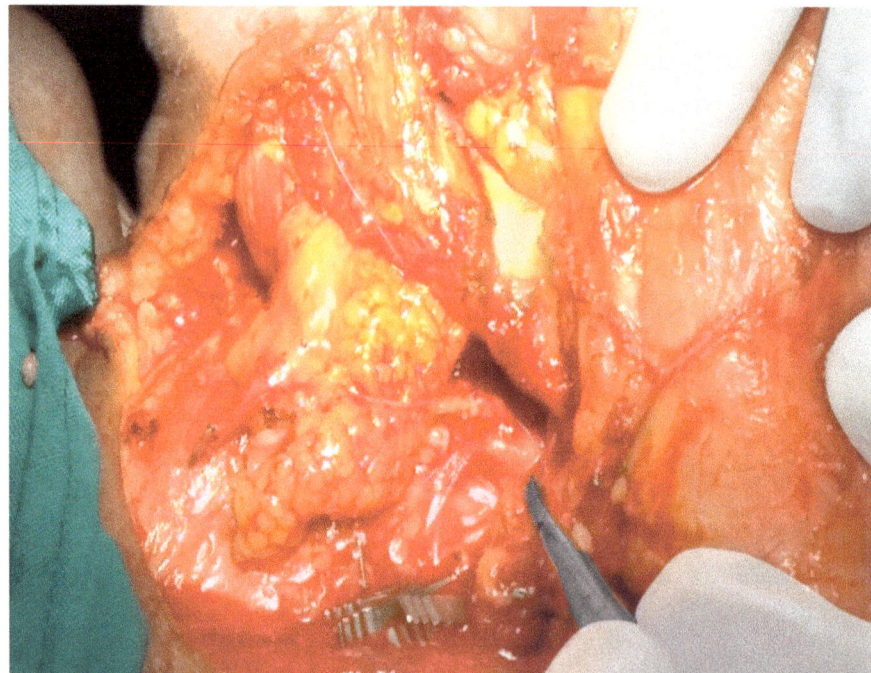

Fig. 73: Lingual nerve is anastomosed with antebrachial nerve for sensation.

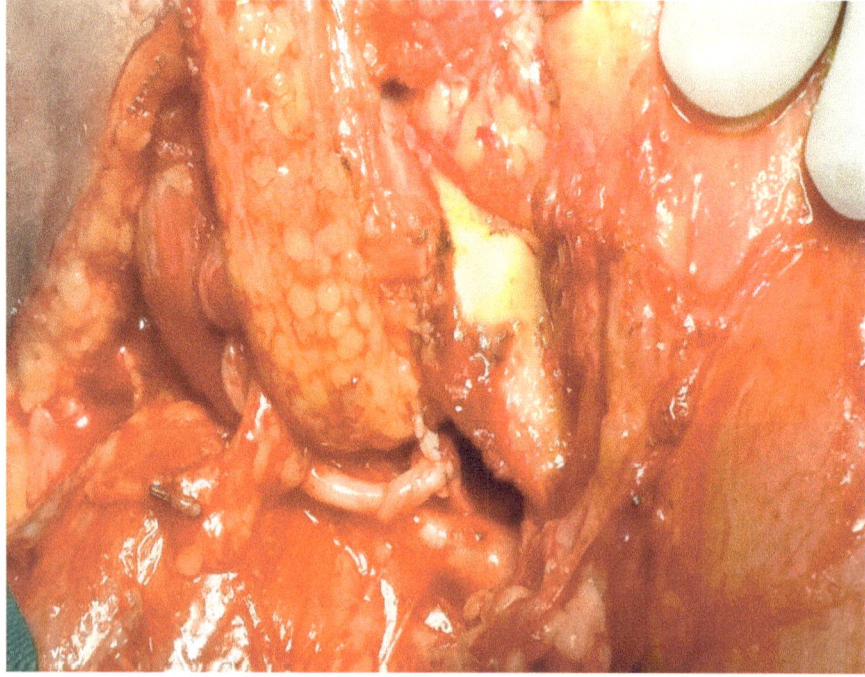

Fig. 74: Nerve is anastomosed with 8-0 prolene.

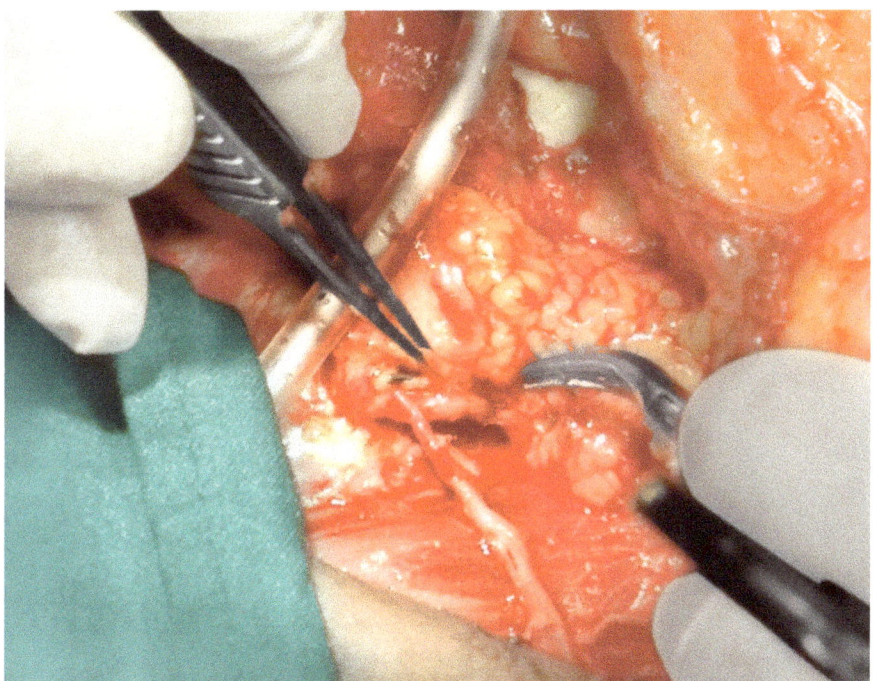

Fig. 75: Radial artery to superior thyroid artery, venae comitant to lingual vein and cephalic vein to external jugular vein anastomoses were done.

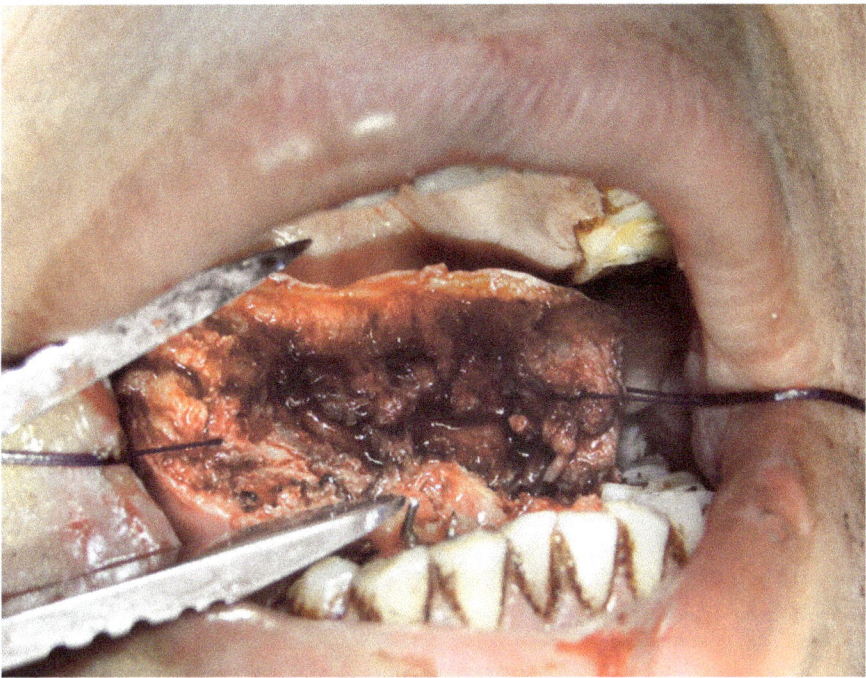

Fig. 76: Total glossectomy is done.[4]

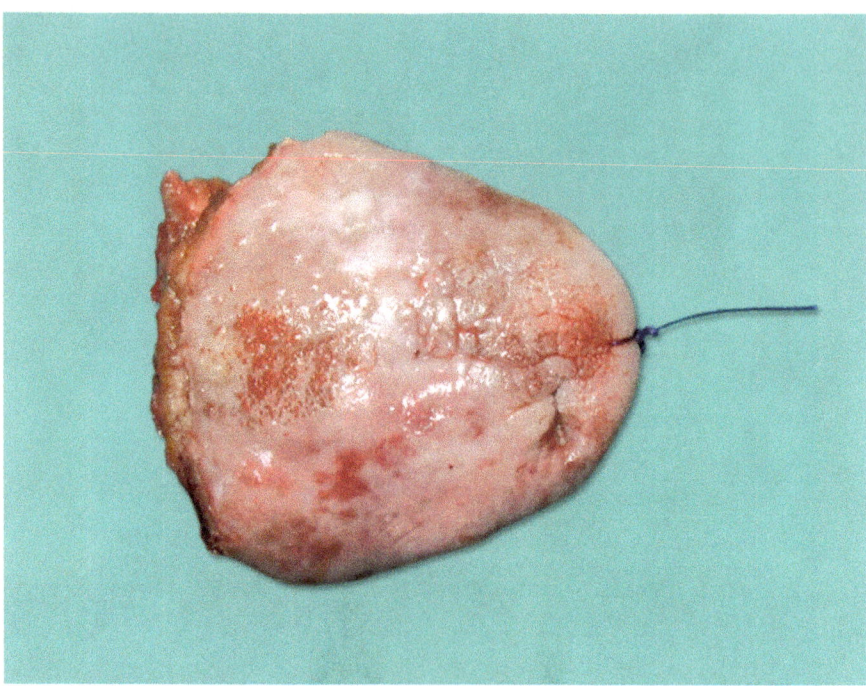

Fig. 77: Excised specimen.

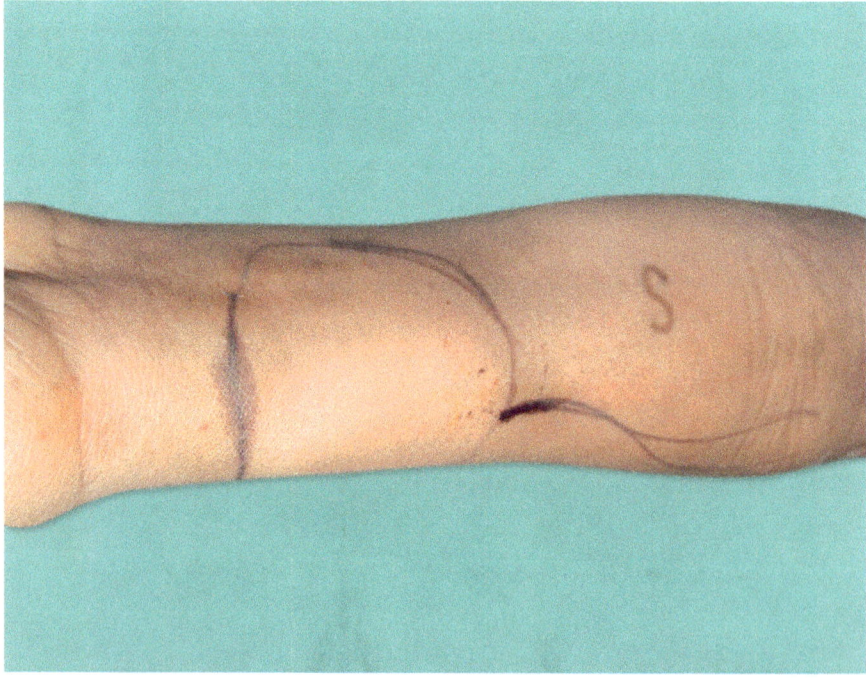

Fig. 78: Marking is done.

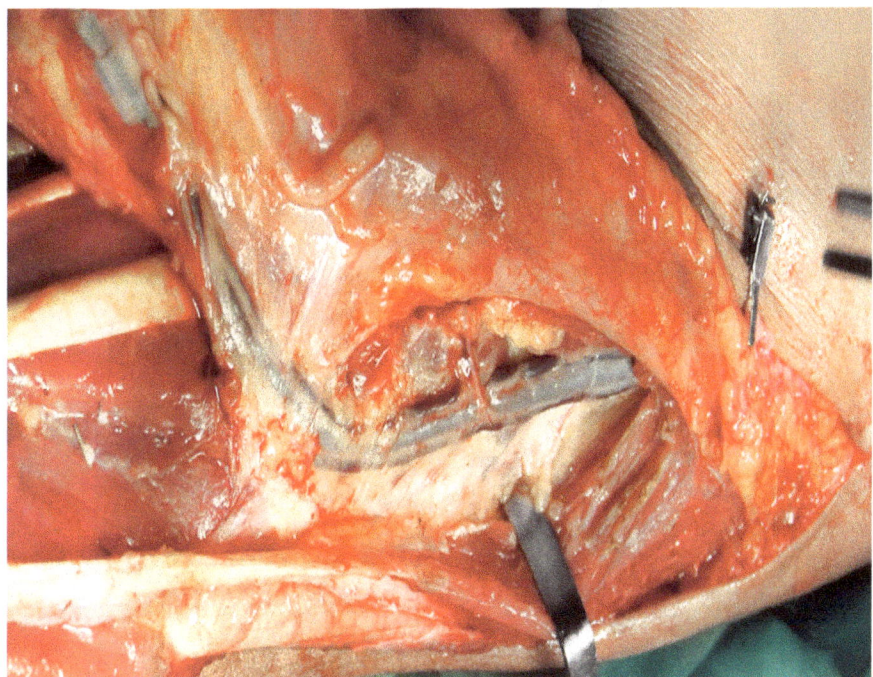

Fig. 79: Flap is raised and pedicle is seen.

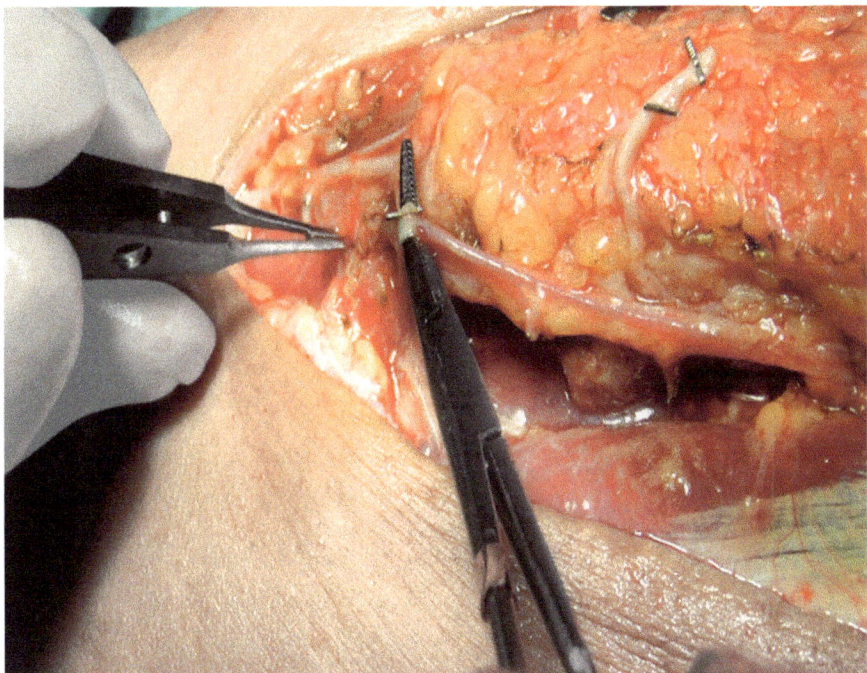

Fig. 80: Venae comitant is seen.

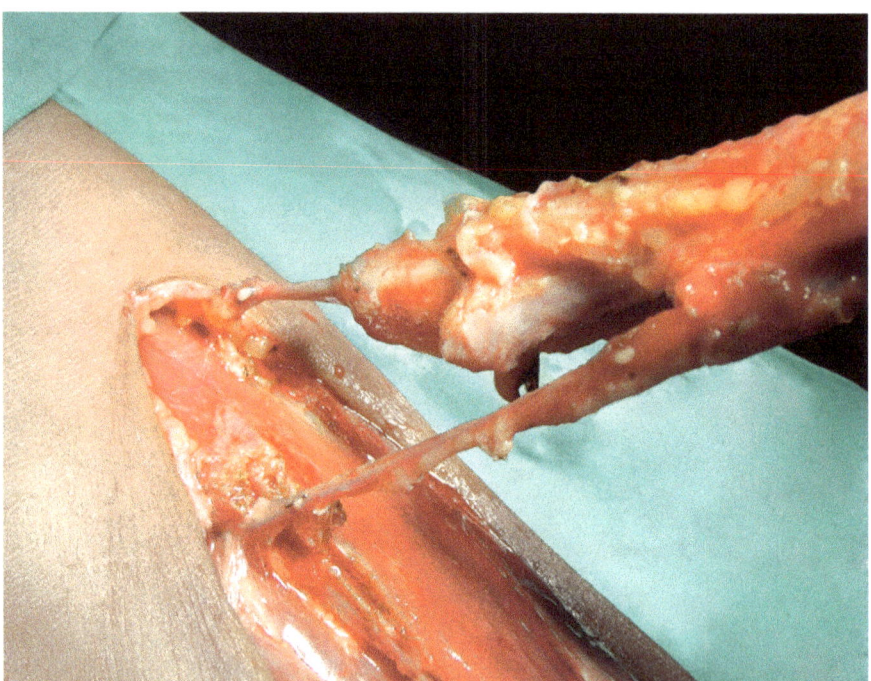

Fig. 81: Flap is raised.

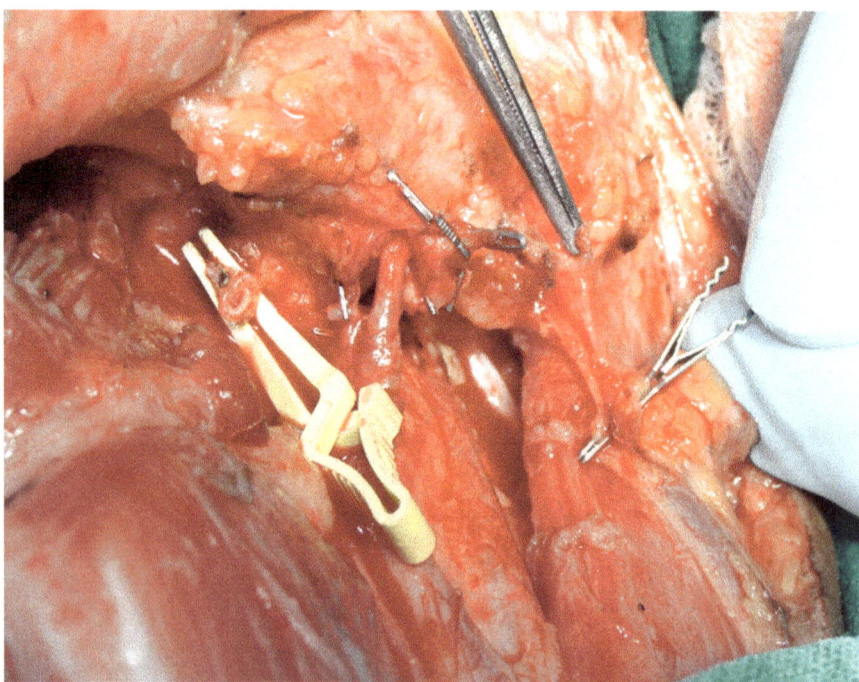

Fig. 82: Vessels are prepared for anastomosis.

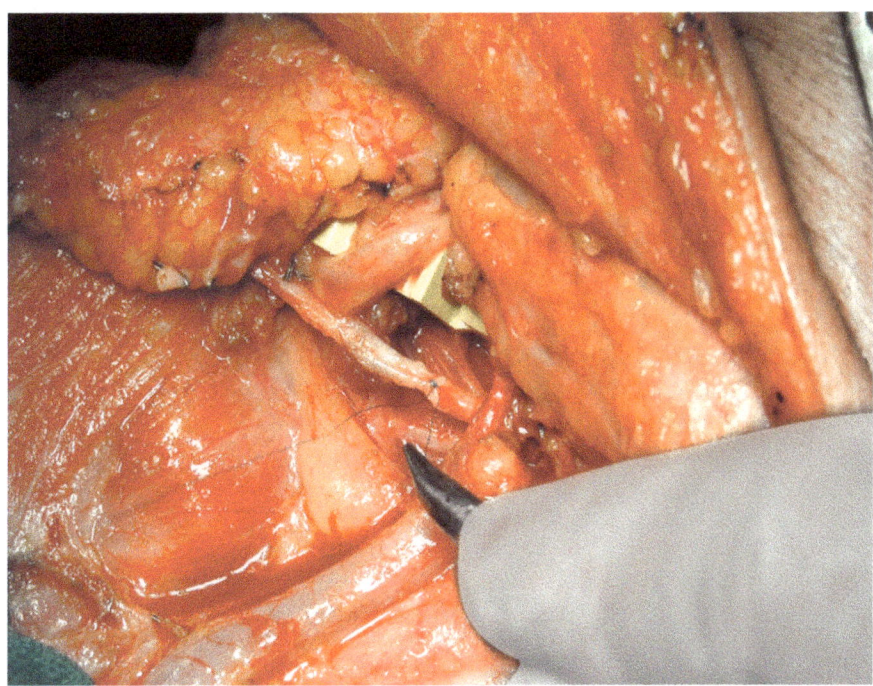

Fig. 83: Lingual nerve is anastomosed to antebrachial nerve.

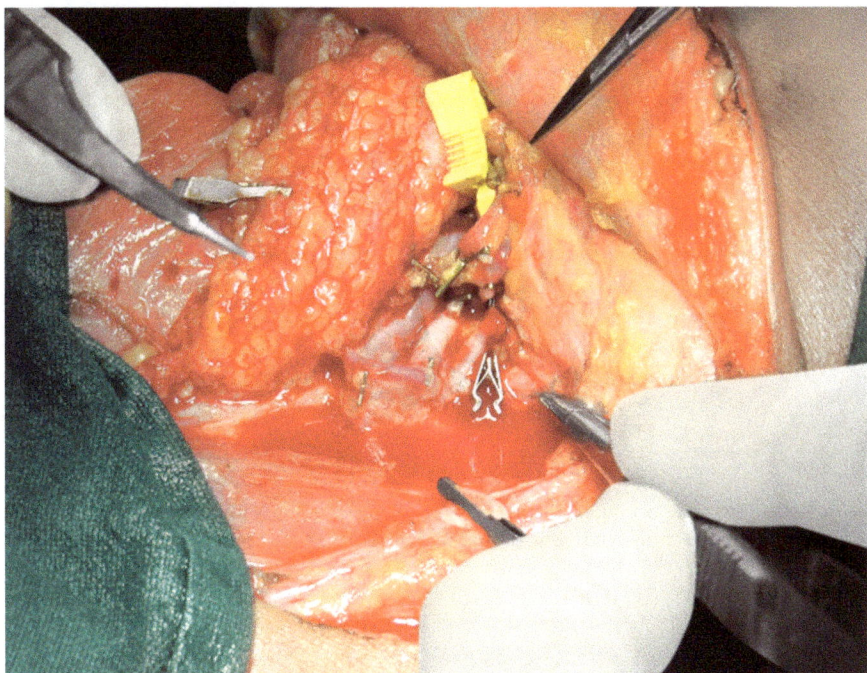

Fig. 84: Radial artery to facial artery, venae comitant to facial vein and cephalic vein to external jugular vein are anastomosed.

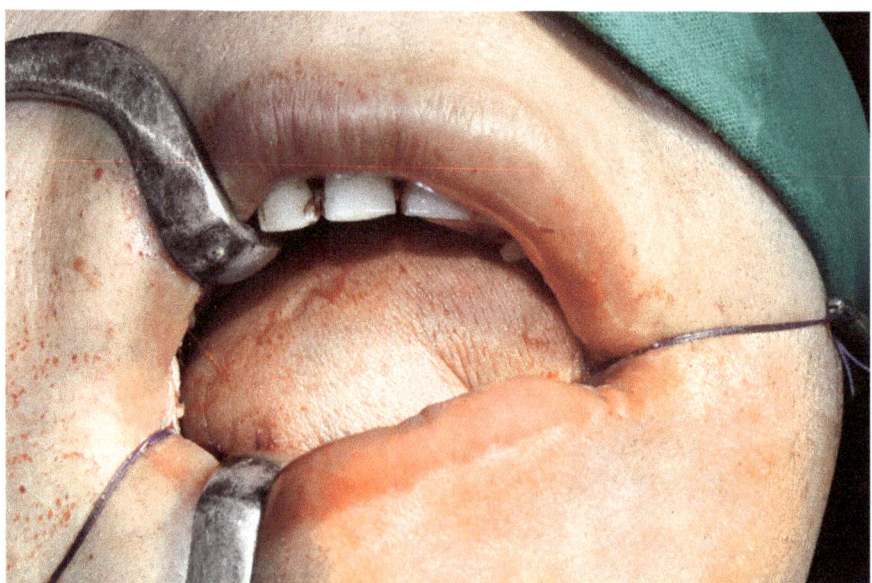

Fig. 85: Inset is completed.

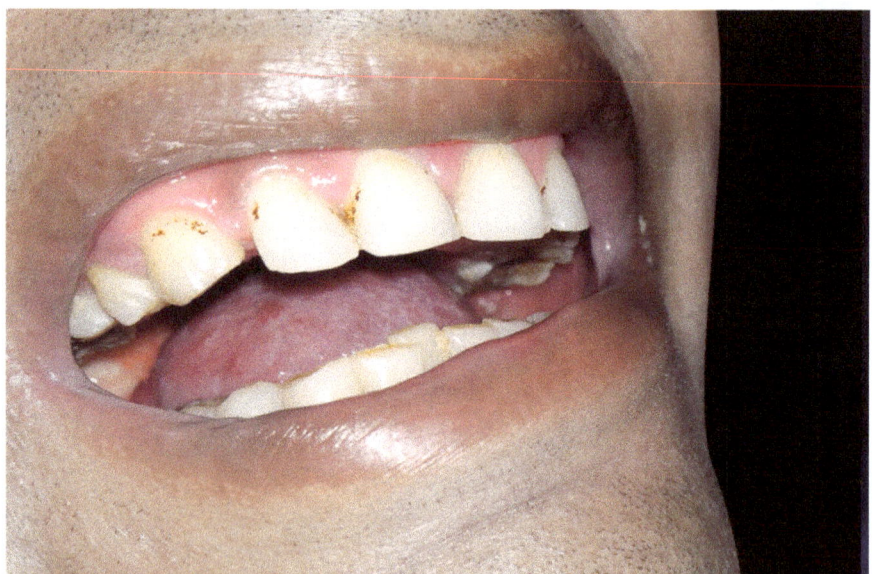

Fig. 86: Patient had good speech and swallowing with adequate functional mobility of the neo-tongue entirely formed by free radial artery forearm flap.

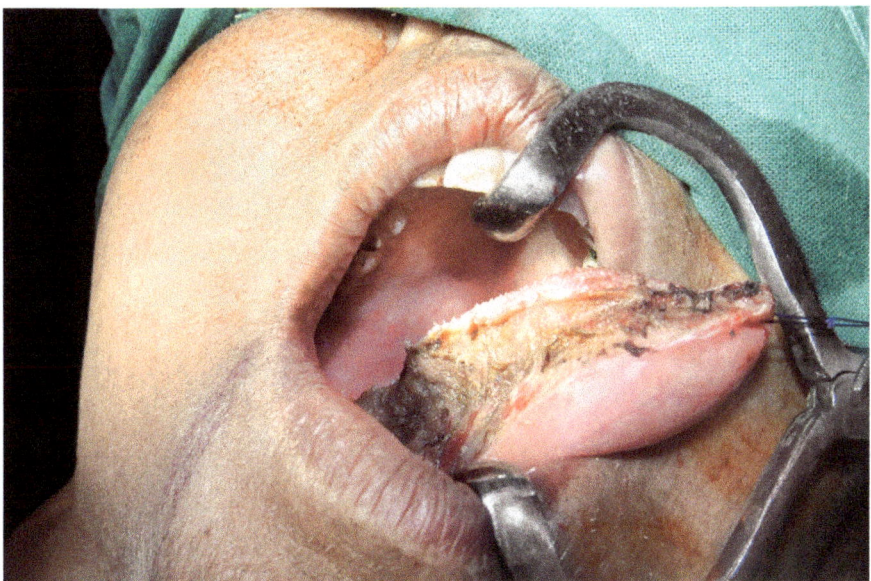
Fig. 87: About 70% of tongue was removed.

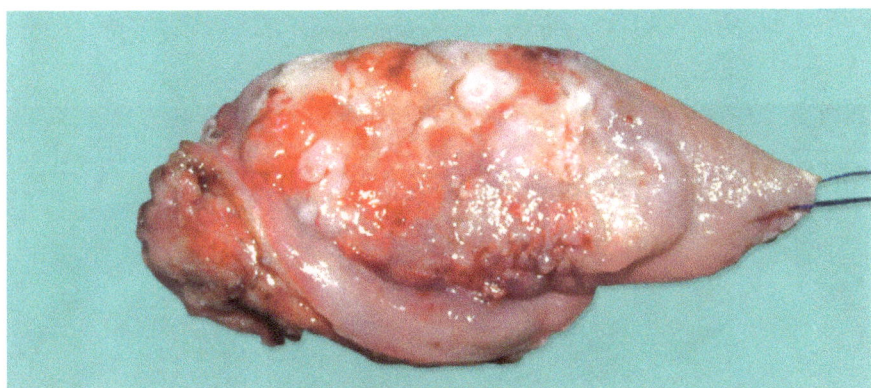
Fig. 88: Excised specimen.

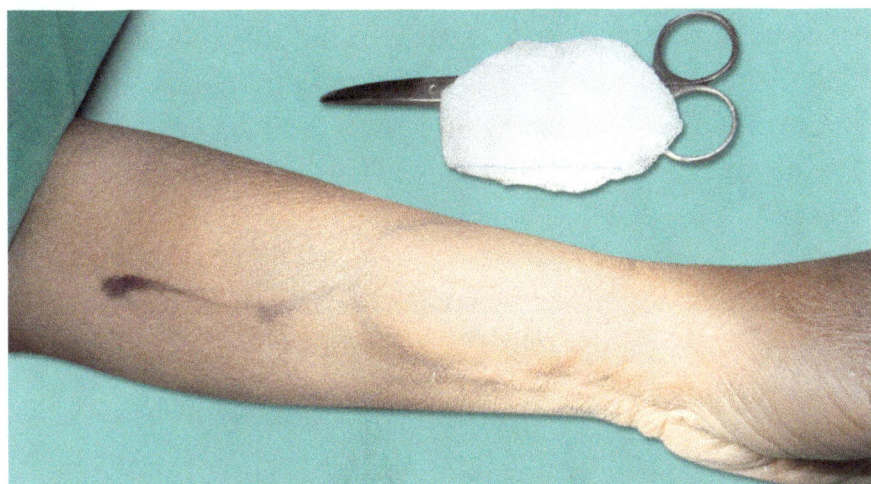
Fig. 89: Measurement and marking were done.

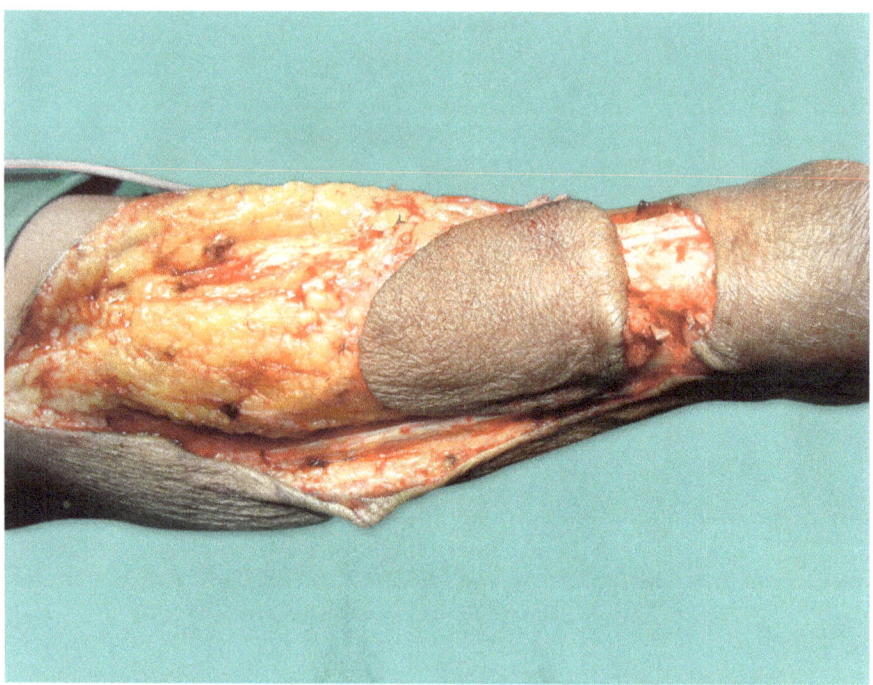

Fig. 90: Flap is being raised.

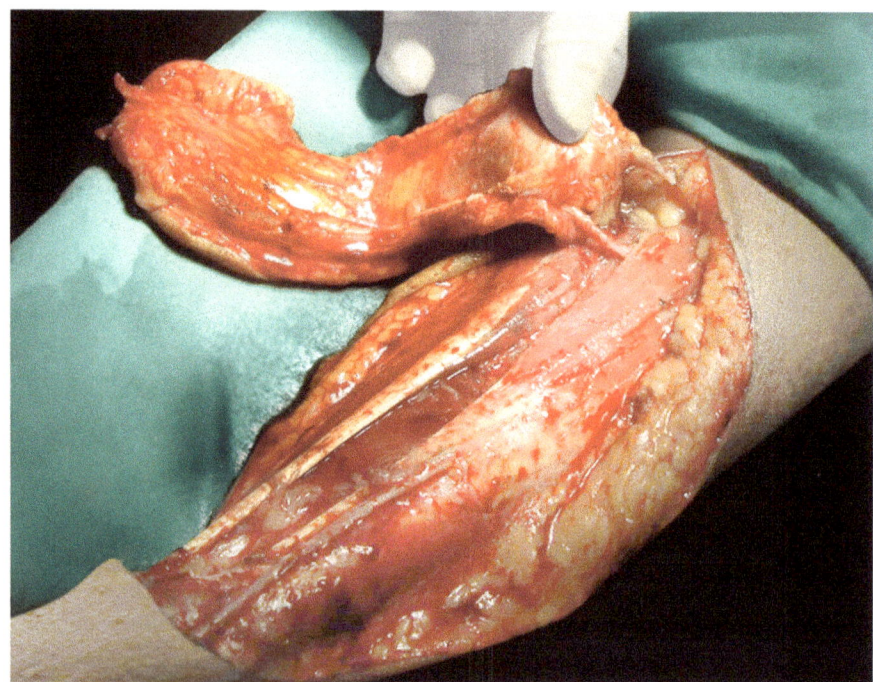

Fig. 91: Flap is elevated.

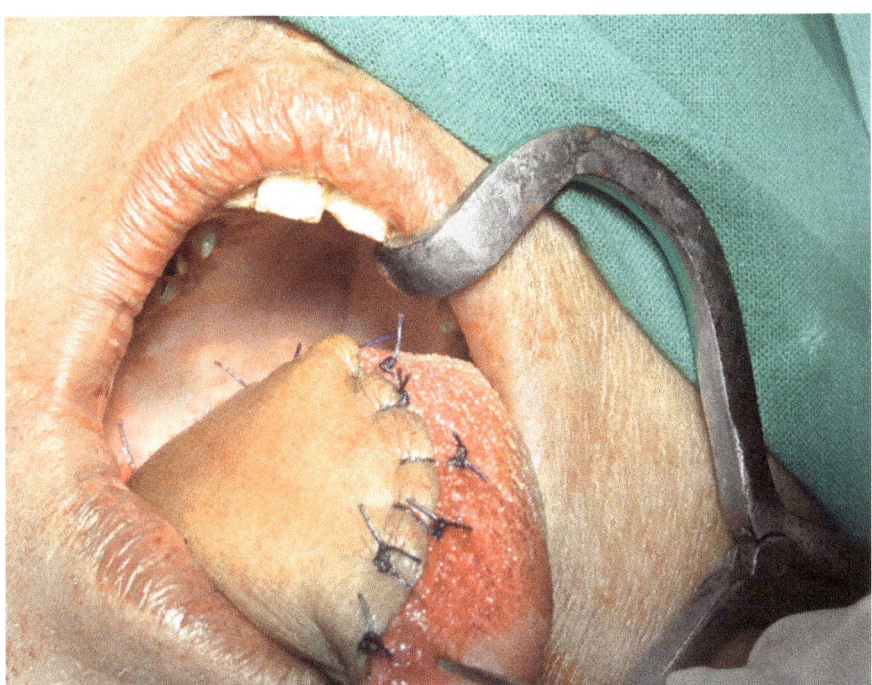

Fig. 92: Inset is completed.

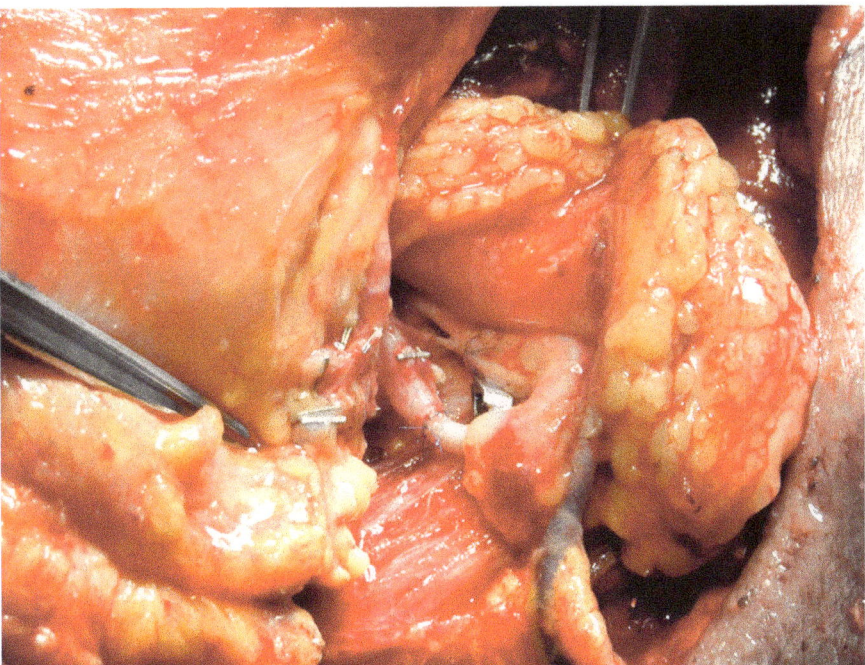

Fig. 93: Lingual nerve is anastomosed to antebrachial nerve and radial artery to facial artery, venae comitant to facial vein and cephalic vein to external jugular vein are anastomosed.

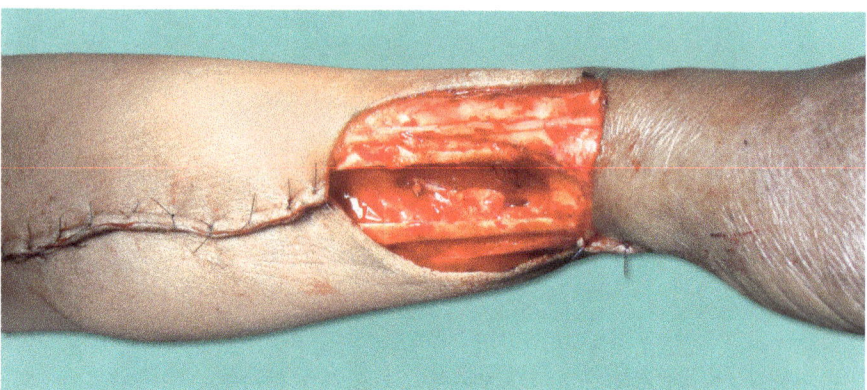

Fig. 94: Donor site.

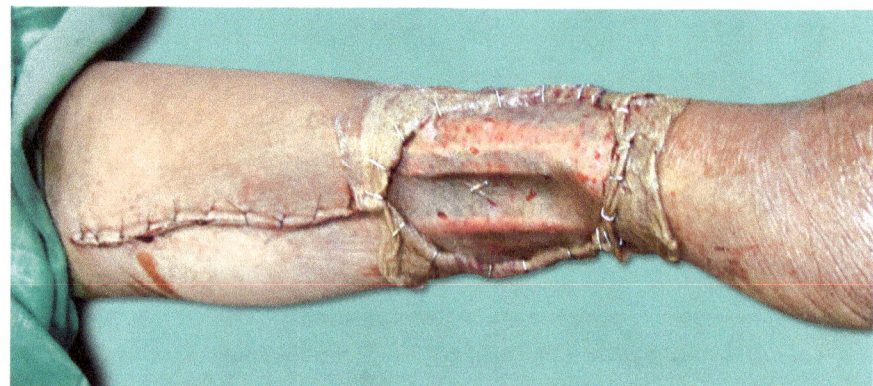

Fig. 95: Donor site is covered with split thickness skin graft.

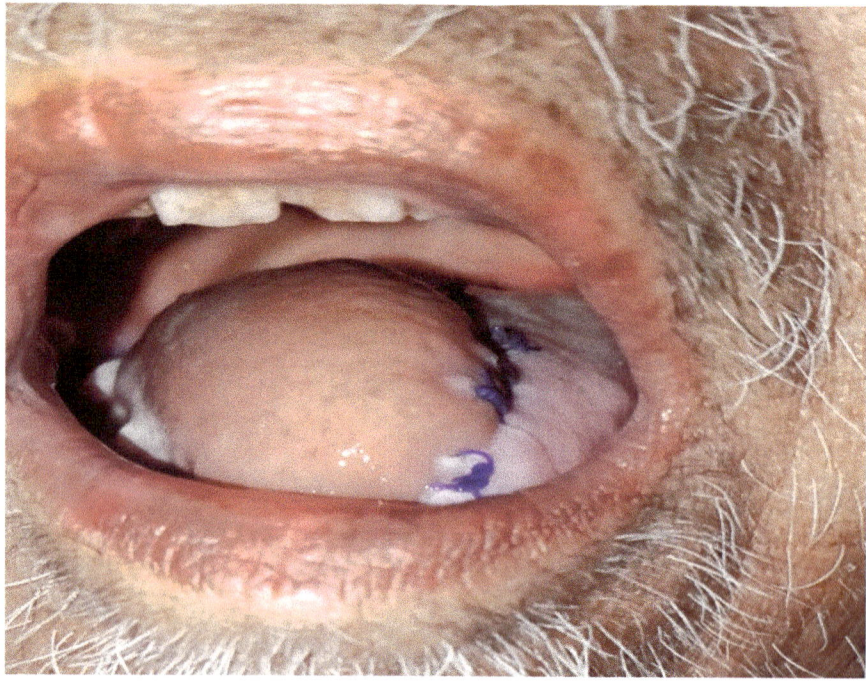

Fig. 96: Postoperative outcome after 20 days.

LONG-TERM FOLLOW-UP CASES

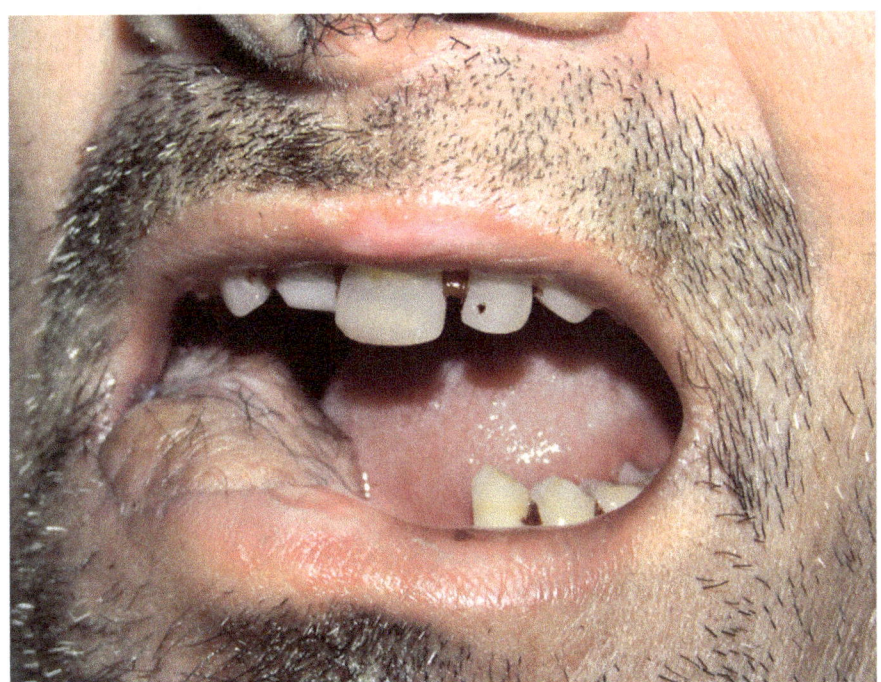

Fig. 97: After 18 months.

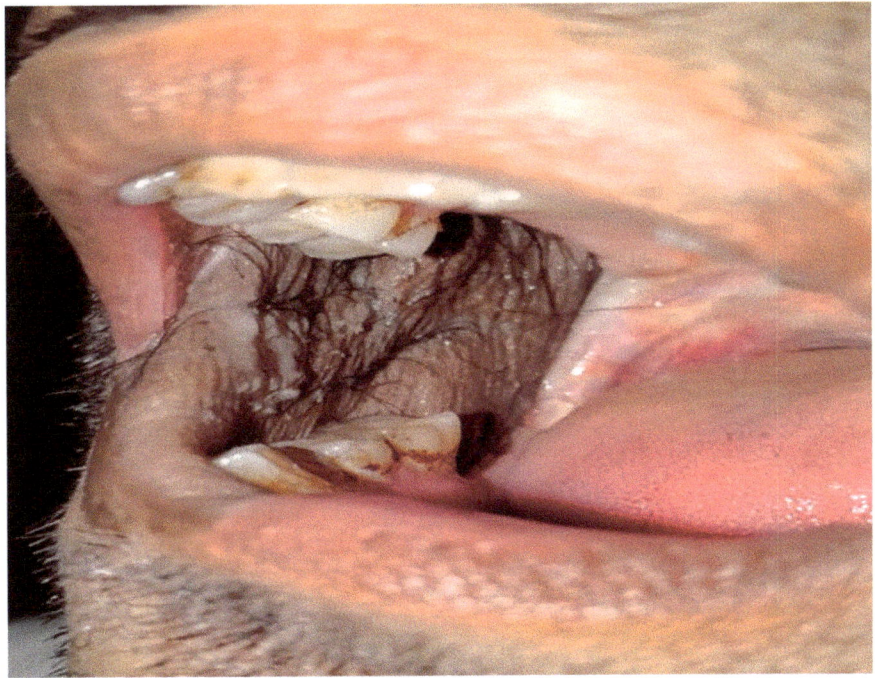

Fig. 98: After 15 months.

REFERENCES

1. Young GF, Chen PJ, Gao YZ, Liu XY, Li J, Jung SH. Forearm skin flap transplantation: a report of 56 cases. J Plast Surg. 1997;50:162-5.
2. Hurvitz KA, Kobayashi M, Evans GR. Current options in head and neck reconstruction. Plast Reconstr Surg. 2006;118:122-33.
3. Hsiao HT, Leu YS, Chang SH, Lee JT. Swallowing function in patients who underwent hemiglossectomy comparison of primary closure and free radial artery forearm flap reconstruction with videofluoroscopy. Ann Plast Surg. 2003;50:450-5.
4. Rhemrev R, Rakhorst HA, Zuidam JM, Mureau MA, Hovius SE, Hofer SO. Long-term functional outcome and satisfaction after radial forearm free flap reconstructions of intraoral malignancy resections. J Plast Reconstr Aesthet Surg. 2007;60:5885-92.

CHAPTER 9

Complications

COMPLICATIONS[1-3]

Free radial artery forearm flap has poor donor site morbidities such as graft loss, exposure of tendons and poor cosmesis of donor site. Patient may develop hematoma in neck requiring re-exploration for hemostasis. Patient may develop partial or total necrosis of flap requiring second surgery.

REFERENCES

1. Lee JW, Jang YC, Oh SJ. Use of the artificial dermis for free radial forearm flap donor site. Ann Plast Surg. 2005;55:500-2.
2. Timmons MJ, Missotten FE, Poole MD, Davies DM. Complications of radial forearm flap donor sites. Br J Plast Surg. 1986;39:176-8.
3. Chen CM, Lin GT, Fu YC, Shieh TY, Huang IY, Shen YS, et al. Complications of free radial forearm flap transfers for head and neck reconstruction. Oral Surg Oral Med Pathol Oral Radiol Endod. 2005;99:671-6.

Suggested Reading

1. Ayer RG, Gupta R. Viragdamania. Mittal shah, Abisheksharma reconstruction of oral neoplasms in indian set up; Redebating the utility of Radial forearm free flaps.http://www.Waent.org/archieves/2010/vol3 -1/20100421 – free-flap- flap.Htm.
2. Becker C, Gilbert A. The cubital flap. Ann Chir Main. 1988;7:136-42.
3. Becker C, Gilbert A. The ulnar flap. Handchir Mikrochir Plast Chir. 1988;20:180-3.
4. Disa JJ, Cordeiro PG, Hidalgo DA. Efficacy of conventional monitoring techniques in free tissue transfer: an 11 years experience in 750 consecutive cases. Plast Reconstr Surg. 1999;104;97-101.
5. Genden EM, Rinaldo A, Suarez C, et al. Complications of free flap transfers for head and neck reconstruction following cancer resection. Oral Oncol. 2004;40;979-84.
6. Gupta S, Jain D, Jhala JT, Saraiya H, Kothari P, Jayesh D, et al. Free radial artery forearm flap I reconstruction of oral cavity cancers our experience. Int J Res Med. 2014;3(4):85-9.
7. Hsiao HT, Leu YS, Chang SH, Lee JT. Swallowing function in patients who underwent hemiglossectomy comparison of primary closure and free radial artery forearm flap reconstruction with videofluoroscopy. Ann Plast Surg. 2003;50:450-5.
8. Hurvitz KA, Kobayashi M, Evans GR. Current options in head and neck reconstruction. Plast Reconstr Surg. 2006;118:122-33.
9. Lee JW, Jang YC, Oh SJ. Esthetic and functional reconstruction for burn deformities of the lower lip and chin with free radial forearm flap. Ann Plast Surg. 2006;56(4):384-6.
10. Markkanen-Leppänen M, Suominen E, Lehtonen H, Asko-Seljavaara S. Free flap reconstructions in the management of oral and pharyngeal cancers. Acta Otolaryngol. 2001;121(3):425-9.
11. Rhemrev R, Rakhorst HA, Zuidam JM, Mureau MA, Hovius SE, Hofer SO. Long-term functional outcome and satisfaction after radial forearm free flap reconstructions of intraoral malignancy resections. J Plast Reconstr Aesthet Surg. 2007;60:5885-92.
12. Santamaria E, Granados M, Barrera-Franco JL. Radial artery forearm flaps for head and neck reconstruction versatility and reliability of a single donor site. Microsurgery. 2000;20:195-201.
13. Weinzweig N, Chen L, Chen ZW. The distally based radial forearm fasciosubcutaneous flap with preservation of the radial artery: an anatomic and clinical approach. Plast Reconstr Surg. 1994;94:675-84.
14. Young GF, Chen PJ, Gao YZ, Liu XY, Li J, Jung SH. Forearm skin flap transplantation: a report of 56 cases. J Plast Surg. 1997;50:162-5.

Index

Page numbers followed by *f* refer to figure.

A

Allen's test 6
    modified 6
Anastomosis, vessels prepared for 76*f*
Antebrachial nerve 1, 7, 77*f*, 81*f*
    lateral 15*f*, 71*f*
Arterial anastomosis 7, 23*f*

B

Bipolar cautery
    dissected with 18*f*
    forceps, fine 10*f*
Brachial artery 4, 7
Brachioradialis 16*f*, 17*f*, 28*f*
    tendons 7
    ulnar border of 15*f*
Buccal mucosa
    carcinoma of 26*f*, 48*f*
    defects of 3
    excision, carcinoma of left 39*f*, 64*f*
    intraoral excision of carcinoma 34*f*

C

Cephalic vein 5, 7, 15*f*, 24*f*, 33*f*, 34*f*, 42*f*, 46*f*, 51*f*, 55*f*, 56*f*, 66*f*, 73*f*, 77*f*, 81*f*
    anatomy of 5, 5*f*
    extended radial to 7
    over radial artery 16*f*
    proximally 14*f*
    thrombosis of 6
    vasculitis of 6
Chemotherapeutic injection causes 6
Chinese flap 2
Cosmetic outcome, excellent 67*f*
Cosmetic result 22*f*
Cubital vein, medial 35*f*

D

Digastric muscle 7, 61*f*
Diploscope 10*f*
Donor site 33*f*, 52*f*, 63*f*, 67*f*, 82*f*
    good cosmetic of 63*f*
Dorsal venous plexus 5

E

Elbow
    dissected up to 14*f*
    dissection
        completed at 19*f*
        of pedicle at 30*f*
    medial cubital vein at 18*f*
    pedicle at 30*f*
    vessels at 36*f*, 49*f*
Excised lesion 12*f*
External jugular vein 7, 20*f*, 33*f*, 51*f*, 56*f*, 62*f*, 66*f*, 77*f*, 81*f*
    anastomoses 73*f*, 42*f*, 46*f*
    with 8-0 prolene 24*f*

F

Facial artery 20*f*, 22*f*, 23*f*, 32*f*, 42*f*, 46*f*, 51*f*, 62*f*, 66*f*, 77*f*, 81*f*
    anastomosed to 56*f*
    proximal part of 7, 61*f*
Facial vein 7, 42*f*, 46*f*, 51*f*, 66*f*, 77*f*, 81*f*
    common 7, 42*f*, 56*f*
    with 10-0 ethilon 32*f*
Fasciocutaneous flap, type C 2
Fingers mouth opening, three and half 68*f*
Flap 80*f*
    subfascial dissection of 17*f*
    total necrosis of 85
Flexor carpi radialis 4, 16*f*, 28*f*
    radial border of 15*f*, 29*f*
    tendon 2, 7
Flexor digitorum superficialis, radial head of 4
Flexor pollicis longus 4
Forearm skin 3
Free radial artery forearm flap 22*f*, 78*f*, 85
    advantages 3
    anatomy 4
    complications 85
    disadvantages 3
    operative steps of 7
    preoperative preparation 6

G

Glossectomy, total 73*f*
Graft loss 85

H

Head and neck resection 1
Hematoma 85
Hemostasis 19*f*, 57*f*
    neck, after 47*f*

I

Incision sutured with 3-0 ethilon 25*f*

J

Jugular vein, internal 7

L

Ligaclip 16*f*
    applicators 9*f*
    ligated with 7
Lingual nerve 70*f*, 72*f*, 77*f*, 81*f*
Lingual vein 7, 73*f*
Low molecular weight dextrose 38
Lower lip
    carcinoma of 48*f*
    excision, carcinoma of 53*f*
    mucosa excision, carcinoma of 58*f*
    support of 55*f*
    with marginal mandibulectomy, carcinoma of 44*f*

M

Mandibulectomy
    marginal 11*f*, 12*f*, 53*f*, 54*f*, 58*f*, 68*f*
    defect after 12*f*
Microsurgery
    clamps for 9*f*
    instruments for 8*f*
Microsurgical reconstruction, instruments for 8

N

Neck dissection and excision, modified 26*f*
Nerve 72*f*
    median 40*f*
Nondominant limb 6

O

Operative microscope 10*f*
Orbicularis oris muscle and flap 56*f*

P

Pad of fat 18*f*
Palmaris longus 1, 55*f*, 56*f*
    tendon 55*f*

Pedicle 17f
Pharyngeal reconstruction 1
Pronator quadratus 4
Pronator teres, attachment of 4

R

Radial artery 4, 32f, 42f, 46f, 51f, 56f, 60f, 62f, 66f, 73f, 77f, 81f
    distally 35f
    forearm flap 1, 2, 4, 6
        drawbacks of 3
    in forearm, anatomy of 4, 4f
    with 8-0 prolene 23f
    with venae comitantes 14f
Radial nerve, sensory branch of 17, 29f
Radius bone 1

S

Saphenous vein graft, interpositional 56f
Sensation, antebrachial nerve for 72f
Sensory radial nerve 17f
    branches of 7
Skin
    graft, split thickness 25f, 33f, 37f, 43f, 52f, 57f, 82f
    paddle, large 3
    thin and pliable 1
Subfascial plane 28f, 29f
Suprafascial dissection 3
Surgical anatomy 4

T

Tendon 61f
Thromboprophylaxis 38

Thyroid
    artery, superior 7, 73f
    vein, superior 7
Tongue reconstruction 1
Tourniquet 7

U

Ulnar artery 4
Upper alveolectomy 39f

V

Venae comitant 18f, 32f, 42f, 46f, 51f, 56f, 60f, 66f, 73f, 75f, 77f, 81f
    to cephalic vein 62f
    to facial vein 62f
Venous anastomosis completed 24f

EU GSPR Authorised Reprsentative
Logos Europe, 9 rue Nicolas Poussin
1700, La Rochelle, France
Phone: +33 (0) 6 67 93 73 78
E-mail: contact@logoseurope.eu

www.ingramcontent.com/pod-product-compliance
Ingram Content Group UK Ltd.
Pitfield, Milton Keynes, MK11 3LW, UK
UKHW051847210426
5322IPUK00019B/293